I0453206

LIFE AFTER

BRAIN

Surgery

ROYSAN SAVINON

Copyright © Year 2025.

All Rights Reserved by Roysan Savinon.

No part of this publication may be reproduced in any form, or by any means, electronic or mechanical, including photocopying, recording, or any information browsing, storage, or retrieval system, without permission in writing from Roysan Savinon.

ISBN

Hardcover: 979-8-90190-076-5

Paperback: 979-8-90190-075-8

Acknowledgments

Hello, everyone. Before we begin this journey together, I want to express my heartfelt gratitude.

First and foremost, I want to express my heartfelt gratitude to my family, my foundation, my support system, and the most incredible gift of all. Words cannot fully convey my appreciation for your unwavering support, love, and encouragement throughout my journey. You have stood by me during my most challenging times, cheering me on, holding my hand, and lifting my spirits when I felt like giving up. With all my heart, I am incredibly grateful to have such a wonderful family. I love you all more than words can express. Thank you for believing in me, for your patience, and for always providing a haven. You are my strength and my daily inspiration.

I appreciate the kindness, support, and constant encouragement from my colleagues and friends, which have helped me keep moving forward. Your uplifting words and belief in my abilities are invaluable to me. I genuinely feel fortunate to have you in my life, and I carry your support with me at every step. Last but not least, I want to sincerely thank the medical team for all the help you have provided.

I want to express my gratitude to my incredible epilepsy community. Thank you for your resilience and courage, and for motivating me to share my story. Your strength reassures me that we are not alone and can shine even brighter together. Your journeys and light inspire me to encourage others and remind everyone that we can all embrace our light, live purposefully, and shine brilliantly regardless of our circumstances.

This book embodies my story and a shared journey filled with hope, resilience, and love. It inspires you to believe in yourself, to persevere through challenges, and to continue shining your light.

I appreciate all of you; thank you for being a part of this incredible journey.

Table of Contents

Chapter 1:
The Start of My Journey

Why I Decided to Share My Experience

Introduction

My epilepsy journey began unexpectedly when I was three years old. I still remember my first seizure, the intense feeling of confusion and fear that overwhelmed me as my body shook and my vision went dark. Although I don't recall all the details, I vividly remember the chaos that followed. My parents' faces still haunt me, their eyes wide with terror, and their voices trembling as they tried to understand what was happening. For them, it was a nightmare they were never prepared for.

The initial seizure was deeply upsetting, not just because of the physical chaos it caused but also because of its symbolic meaning: a sudden break in our otherwise stable environment, a moment when life's simple, valuable nature was unexpectedly shattered. The questions that raced through my mind: What is happening? Will he recover? Is this forever? highlight the uncertainty and fear that come with such an event. Seeing their child suffer from this invisible illness without a full understanding to explain or reassure left a profound impact on me, sparking a deep emotional reaction.

Subsequently, my life was irrevocably altered. As time progressed, the frequency of seizures increased, each seeming like an unpredictable upheaval, an uncontrollable storm that could emerge unexpectedly at any moment.

Doctors ran numerous tests, including EEG scans, MRIs, and bloodwork, to find out what was causing my condition. I faced numerous appointments, consultations, and reassurances that I would have an uncertain future. My parents clung to hope, but I could see the worry and despair behind their brave faces. Eventually, I was diagnosed with epilepsy, a diagnosis that would cast a long shadow over my life. At first, it felt like a permanent sentence, a condition that would define my days. We were told I'd need medication forever, and while the meds helped reduce the frequency and severity of my seizures, they also caused side effects, fatigue, mood swings, and foggy periods that made me feel disconnected from myself. It seemed I might never fully escape this reality, that my future would always be shaped by these invisible storms.

However, I have come to realize a fundamental truth: even when healthcare professionals delineate certain limitations, life possesses an inherent unpredictability that can open new opportunities. No individual can fully prepare for such experiences, particularly as a child navigating life with a chronic condition in a world that often appears to move too swiftly, leaving one behind. The profound fear and affection of my parents transformed into a multitude of questions; their intentions were to protect me and ensure my safety. Nonetheless, the pervasive uncertainty infiltrated every aspect of our existence. Their hearts were burdened by the sight of my ordeal, yet they steadfastly refused to allow despair to define our journey.

That moment marked the commencement of a lifelong journey not solely for myself but for my entire family unit. What ensued was a whirlwind of medical consultations, examinations, treatments, and continual assessments. Each new specialist and medication brought with them hope and uncertainty. We acquired the ability to interpret medical jargon critically and to advocate vigorously for answers. Over time, I confronted the stark reality: epilepsy was a component of my narrative; however, it did not have to define the entirety of it.

It constituted a chapter and a challenge, but not the conclusion. Living with epilepsy necessitated adjustments to our daily routines, more meticulous planning, constant vigilance, and an enhanced awareness of my limitations and vulnerabilities.

We mourn the loss of an envisioned future, one devoid of fears, abundant in spontaneous adventures, and carefree days. This was the loss we lamented: the innocence of childhood dreams that suddenly felt distant. Nevertheless, as the years progressed, I recognized that amidst this loss, a new chapter was emerging, one of growth, strength, and resilience. We understood that although epilepsy might influence certain aspects of life, it did not define my spirit or my potential. It became evident that even in the face of uncertainty, there remained space for hope, determination, and a meaningful life.

My goal in sharing my story is to let others know you are not alone in your struggles. Whether you're dealing with a chronic condition, emotional pain, or life-changing circumstances, there is hope. It's a journey of adapting and building resilience, one where, even amid challenges, you can discover new strengths and redefine what's possible. My message is simple: Your story is still being written. Even when the future seems uncertain, remember that every moment of hardship offers potential for growth.

This story transcends mere limitations; it's a tribute to the human spirit that refuses to give up, constantly searches for light in the darkness, and rises each day with courage. If you're on this journey right now, know that I'm here to support you by sharing my own experiences so you can see for yourself. *The emotional journey includes grief, acceptance, and growth.*

Receiving an epilepsy diagnosis can be like grieving a part of life that's lost. As I got older and understood what epilepsy meant, I felt like I was falling behind my peers. I longed to be like other kids, carefree and spontaneous, without a care in the world. But instead, I had to deal with medication schedules, limitations, hospital trips, and unpredictable moments of vulnerability that could hit me at any moment.

I felt different sometimes, and other times, I felt broken.

There were times when I felt like I was drifting away from everything around me. Other days, I felt like I was at the end of my rope, burdened by doubts and fears that seemed too much to handle. But during those tough moments, my family was my rock. They kept me grounded, protecting me from falling deeper into darkness. Their unwavering love was a beacon that helped me find my way when I thought I had nothing left.

My siblings, extended family, and close friends didn't just stand by; they were my companions every step of the way, even when things were uncertain. Having them around brought moments of joy, laughter, and a sense of normalcy when everything else felt chaotic. They helped me through my physical, emotional, and mental wounds, and reminded me that I was still connected to life and to others. Their support didn't just lift my spirits; it reinforced the truth that I believe in you're never truly alone in your struggles. Looking back, I feel an overwhelming sense of gratitude, especially to God, who has blessed me with such a caring and unwavering family and loved ones.

Their unwavering support has served as a fundamental source of strength, guiding me through challenging days, prolonged nights, and times when my hopes waned. Their love stands as a testament to the significance of community and the profound power of solidarity in the face of life's adversities. I am sharing this because I believe many individuals, particularly within the epilepsy community, will resonate with their own experiences reflected here.

Living with a condition that fluctuates unpredictably can feel isolating, and it can sometimes make you question your worth. However, I wish to remind you that support, particularly from those who genuinely understand, is invaluable. It serves as the foundation that can help you rebuild, restart, and reclaim your sense of purpose. For this reason, I have opted to share my story not to focus on hardships, but to emphasize hope grounded in perseverance and the resilience of the human spirit.

Even when the going gets tough, there's always a light that can show us the way. For many of you reading this, you'll see your own experiences reflected here, moments of fear, breakthroughs that came from pain, and a relentless drive to live life to the fullest. My heartfelt hope is that these words inspire you to keep moving forward, to persevere, and to have faith in your own extraordinary potential. Remember, you're not alone. Epilepsy doesn't define who you are.

It's just one piece of your story, a chapter that, with courage, can become a powerful tale of resilience. You can lead a vibrant life filled with energy, positivity, and purpose. That might seem ambitious, but I've seen firsthand that even in the face of unpredictability and setbacks, we can find strength, joy, and meaning. I know many people view epilepsy as a limitation.

There have been occasions when I have experienced feelings of entrapment, akin to my condition hindering me from realizing my full potential. This is a common sentiment; everyone encounters moments when they perceive their circumstances as insurmountable. However, I wish to offer encouragement: do not let a constrained mindset become an obstacle. Our capabilities often extend far beyond our own perceptions or the beliefs of others.

More than just a memoir, this book is a powerful tribute to hope and the human spirit's resilience. For those living with epilepsy, daily challenges include unpredictable seizures, fear of the unknown, and often a deep sense of loneliness. However, it also highlights the importance of perseverance, faith, and the inner strength that drives us. It shows how resilient we are able to bounce back after a fall, find purpose amid chaos, and turn adversity into opportunities for growth. Most importantly, I want you to know that your story matters.

Too many of us have kept our true selves hidden, locked away by shame, fear, or the fear that nobody will understand. I've been there too. I kept quiet about my struggles for years, thinking that sharing my story would make me seem weak or a burden to others. But I've come to realize something important: many people are quietly battling similar challenges. They need to hear, through your story, that they're not alone. That's why I'm opening up about my own journey.

This is intended for individuals living with epilepsy; however, it also addresses those who feel confined, whether due to circumstances, self-doubt, or societal expectations. It is for parents who feel powerless, teenagers overwhelmed by shame, and adults trapped in routines they no longer wish to follow. Furthermore, it is for caregivers, siblings, and friends who support others and often bear unseen burdens themselves.

In the forthcoming chapters, I intend to explore my extensive experience with epilepsy surgery, a procedure often regarded as a last resort or a significant leap of faith. While not every individual with epilepsy qualifies as a potential candidate for surgery, and I will address the realistic factors involved, my goal is that my narrative provides insight, hope, and encouragement.

An Unexpected Opportunity for Growth

Although epilepsy was once seen as a limitation, a constant barrier that restricted my freedom and cast doubt over every part of my life, it gradually became a crucible, a space where my true strength, patience, and understanding were developed. Looking back on this experience, I realize that my condition compelled me to develop qualities that many people spend years cultivating: emotional resilience, self-awareness, and the ability to adapt quickly to unexpected challenges.

From an early age, I was compelled to attentively monitor my body, recognizing warning signals, understanding the sensations linked to my seizures, and discerning when to seek assistance or adopt precautionary measures. I have developed the ability to advocate for myself within medical environments, posing questions, obtaining second opinions, and making informed decisions regarding treatment options and lifestyle modifications. Requesting assistance from family, friends, or healthcare professionals was not always straightforward; however, it became an essential aspect of my personal development. This process instilled humility, trust, and an appreciation for community support. In numerous respects, epilepsy accelerated my maturation beyond that of my peers.

As I faced health challenges, I also became more empathetic and better attuned to the pain, perseverance, and quiet struggles of others. I saw the unseen battles fought behind closed doors and learned firsthand the importance of patience and kindness. Over the years, my experiences have shaped my outlook, turning hardship into a gift that has given me empathy, strengthened my faith, and made me more grateful for each moment of life.

With that perspective, I now see my condition as more than just a challenge; it's a teacher that has given me valuable lessons about resilience, vulnerability, and hope. It's made me more compassionate, helped me connect with others on a deeper level, and given me a sense of purpose: to share my story, support those on a similar path, and remind everyone that strength can come from struggle. Today, I want to say to you: I see you, I understand you, and you're stronger than you think.

Let's now embark on a thorough exploration of the intricacies involved in the journey.

I understand that the idea of brain surgery can cause feelings of being overwhelmed and very distressing for many people. Just hearing about "brain surgery" can trigger waves of fear, uncertainty, or anxiety, which are completely normal since the brain is, after all, the most important organ in the human body. Thinking about such a procedure can be overwhelming, especially when the stakes are high and there are many unknowns.

I want to reassure you that you're not alone in feeling this way. Many people have faced similar fears, and these feelings are valid, natural, and an important part of the decision-making process when considering such a life-changing procedure.

Before my own surgery in February 2021, I was overwhelmed with intense emotions. I remember the days leading up to the operation, each hour filled with a mix of hope, anxiety, and many questions. I felt a deep sense of dread, worried about possible complications during the procedure. I wondered what unexpected events might occur. The prospect of unforeseen issues stayed on my mind, making me wonder: Is the risk worth it? Will I fully recover? These thoughts kept spinning in my head, creating a never-ending cycle of "what if" scenarios that disturbed my sleep and made my heart race.

Some days, I felt like I was going to jump out of my skin with anxiety, stuck in the silent, sterile hospital room, staring at the ceiling, feeling scared and uncertain about what was next. The worried looks from my family, their whispered hopes, and their quiet prayers only made my own fears worse. The weight of their concern made me realize how deeply this decision was affecting everyone around me, not just me. But despite all these emotions, I knew deep down that staying stuck in that fear wouldn't help me make the best decision or move toward healing. As time passed, I discovered that focusing on hope and the possibility of a better life was crucial.

Every day, I reminded myself that brain surgery, despite being complex and intimidating, is typically a carefully planned and precise procedure performed by some of the world's most skilled neurosurgeons. These experts dedicate their lives to understanding the brain, utilizing the latest technology, thorough evaluations, and teamwork to achieve the safest possible outcomes. Choosing to move forward wasn't a decision I took lightly. It involved extensive evaluations, including scans, tests, and consultations with multiple doctors who thoroughly examined my case from every angle.

My medical team reviewed my medical history, weighed the risks, and walked me through the procedure step by step, emphasizing that it was tailored to my specific needs. I developed trust in them. Their professionalism, compassion, and honesty made me feel more at ease and less like I was embarking on something unfamiliar. I stayed open-minded and committed to the process, knowing the decision was driven by a desire to enhance my quality of life.

Neurosurgery can be life-changing. For me, it has significantly reduced the frequency and severity of my seizures, giving me a newfound sense of freedom and hope. I now live a life that was once just a dream. It could provide the same opportunities for others considering this procedure.

Nevertheless, it is crucial to recognize that such a decision should not be made hastily. Each person's circumstances differ, and a solution that works for one individual may not be appropriate for another. Therefore, I strongly recommend consulting a qualified neurologist or epilepsy specialist. These experts are trained to conduct thorough evaluations, discuss the associated risks and benefits, and help you make an informed decision based on your specific situation.

As I move forward, I'll be sharing my personal journey, from preparing my mind and emotions to undergoing surgery and rebuilding my life. By sharing my story, I aim to demonstrate that even when the path feels tough or uncertain, there's always hope, support, and the opportunity for a brighter future. It's essential to remember that you're not alone. Please reach out to trusted healthcare providers, gather all the necessary information, and stay positive. Taking that brave first step can lead to incredible changes in your life.

A Comprehensive Exploration of Shadows and Light: My Journey with Epilepsy

At that time, I was merely a child, too young to fully comprehend the events unfolding around me, yet sufficiently aware to sense the profound fear that gripped me whenever shadows encroached. My recollections of the initial seizure are vague, as I was too young and frightened, which has rendered my memories somewhat hazy. However, the accounts shared by my family regarding that day continue to resonate with me: the fear, the panic, and the helplessness they experienced as they watched their young daughter lose control.

That moment marked the beginning of a lifelong struggle, one that tested my body, mind, and spirit; yet, over time, it also revealed strengths I never knew I possessed. As the years passed, my seizures became more frequent, creeping into my daily life like unwelcome shadows, unpredictable, uninvited, and often overwhelming. Sometimes, I'd be doing something ordinary, playing with friends, doing homework, or just lying in bed, and suddenly, darkness would wash over me, leaving me exhausted and disoriented. It felt like being trapped inside my own body, a place where frustration, exhaustion, and feelings of misunderstanding became constant companions.

Despite daily challenges, I endeavored to maintain a semblance of normalcy, notwithstanding the seizures that rendered such an effort seemingly unattainable. I vividly remember the tranquil mornings when I would awaken, harboring hopes for a different outcome, only to confront the stark reality of my condition. I questioned myself with inquiries for which I often lacked answers: Will this situation ever improve? Will I perpetually feel this way? While medications aided in managing some seizures, they never achieved complete control. At times, I experienced a sensation akin to walking a tightrope, oscillating between hope and despair, aware that I was exerting all possible effort, yet overwhelmed by the burden of uncertainty.

There were days when I felt so frustrated that I'd lash out, cry silently, or crash into exhaustion after an episode. It was exhausting both emotionally and physically. The idea of surgery came up as a possible solution, a way to take back control and get my life back. I still remember how the room fell silent when I first heard the words "brain surgery." It was as if the air had been sucked out, and my heart began racing with fear and uncertainty. I was flooded with questions. Was I really ready for this? And the weight of that decision was crushing me.

In the weeks preceding the surgery, I struggled internally with a tumult of doubts. I contemplated whether the risk was justified, questioned the possibility of unforeseen complications, and wondered about the completeness of my recovery. The fear at times proved paralyzing, leading me to question my resilience. I recall nights spent awake, gazing at the ceiling, with tears tracing down my cheeks as I grappled with uncertainty.

The future seemed bleaker and more uncertain than ever before. However, amidst this emotional upheaval, I also maintained a sense of hope. I permitted myself to envision a life beyond seizures, one in which I could breathe freely, pursue my ambitions unimpeded, and restore my independence. I persisted in believing that this surgical procedure could serve as a pivotal moment, a chance to redefine my life narrative. The day of the operation was characterized by a tumult of emotions: fear, anticipation, and a glimmer of hope.

The procedure was not an immediate remedy, and I recognized that recovery would require time. Following the surgery, I faced various challenges, including extended recovery periods, adjustments to medication, and occasional frustrations stemming from perceived slow progress. However, the advancements I have achieved since then are noteworthy: my seizures have become less frequent and less severe, and I feel as though I am beginning to truly live rather than merely endure.

Reflecting on my experience, I am overwhelmed with a profound sense of gratitude. I extend my sincere appreciation to the exceptional medical team, including surgeons, nurses, and specialists, whose expertise and compassionate care facilitated my recovery. I also acknowledge those who stood by me, providing encouragement and love during my most vulnerable moments. Above all, I am indebted for the inner strength I have uncovered that quiet, persistent voice affirming, "You can do this," even amid doubt.

This journey has imparted upon me that even during our most challenging moments, hope and resilience can develop quietly, guiding us through adversity. It serves as a reminder that, regardless of how insurmountable circumstances may appear, our capacities are greater than we often acknowledge. Living with epilepsy has been an integral part of my narrative; however, it does not define my identity. Instead, it has become a chapter characterized by resilience, courage, and hope, one that continues to evolve with each new day.

I share my account to convey to others that they are not alone, whether confronting epilepsy, a health challenge, or other difficulties.

Share My Story with You

If you're reading this and struggling with epilepsy or any mental health issue, you're not alone. Whether you're just coming to terms with your diagnosis, thinking about treatment or surgery, or feeling overwhelmed by the uncertainty of what's to come, I want you to know: You're not alone, and your worth isn't defined by your condition. Living with epilepsy can be incredibly tough. It can sometimes feel like a weight, a hurdle, or a limitation, especially when seizures disrupt school, work, or daily life.

I have encountered those instances, days when I felt confined within my own body, distressed by the inability to perform actions I previously took for granted. The apprehension that a seizure might occur at any time, or that my future could be constrained, can exert considerable emotional and mental burden. However, the truth I have come to realize through my personal journey is that epilepsy constitutes merely one chapter in one's life, not the entirety of the story. It can impart unforeseen lessons in resilience, compassion, patience, and faith. It can also serve as a reminder that even in our most vulnerable moments, an inner strength awaits emergence.

I firmly believe that we possess greater courage and perseverance than we often give ourselves credit for. Reflecting on my experiences, I realize that I have overcome considerably more than I initially perceived: days marked by doubt, nights spent contemplating the future, and moments of feeling powerless. Nonetheless, with each day, I discovered support, information, and hope. Being surrounded by compassionate healthcare professionals, loving family members, and a community sharing similar struggles was essential. Accurate information regarding my condition helped dispel myths and fears, thereby providing a clearer path forward. I wish to underscore the importance of understanding that hope and healing are indeed attainable. Despite the waves of fear, frustration, and uncertainty, life persists, and it can be fulfilling, joyful, and purposeful.

I am aware of this through direct observation of how resilience develops in the most unforeseen circumstances. Whether it involves garnering strength from minor achievements such as controlling a seizure or handling a challenging appointment or fostering patience during extended recovery periods, every progression is significant. To all individuals experiencing fear or doubt, I extend my sincere understanding and compassion. I have been in your position, I have endured sleepless nights, anxiety, and moments when surrender appeared more accessible. However, I have learned that even amidst these difficulties, a glimmer of hope persists, ready to be ignited by courage and support.

Keep in mind that a bright future is waiting for you beyond epilepsy. It might not be exactly what you pictured, and the path may be full of twists and turns, but it's within your grasp. Your journey is one-of-a-kind, but your strength is something we all share. When you're surrounded by love, accurate information, and a faith in your own resilience, obstacles start to become stepping stones.

So, let's embark on this journey together with hope for tomorrow, the courage to face today, and the unwavering belief that a better future is always within reach. Your story is still unfolding, and I truly believe that even in the midst of challenges, hope will guide your way. You're stronger than you think, and a life full of purpose, meaning, and possibility is waiting for you just ahead.

When times got tough, I discovered a deep well of strength within myself, thanks to the unwavering love of my family. Their encouragement became my anchor: my parents' gentle guidance, the patience of my loved ones during my hospital stays, and their quiet faith in my potential gave me the push I needed to keep going when I felt like giving up. I'll always be grateful to God for providing me with such a caring and supportive network. Their presence served as a powerful reminder that I wasn't alone in this fight. As the seizures continued, the option of surgery was discussed.

I recall that day with vivid clarity; the atmosphere abruptly became oppressive, and my heartbeat quickened amidst a blend of hope and anxiety. The reference to "brain surgery" bore considerable significance. I pondered the possibility of losing more than I would gain, contemplating the associated risks, the recovery process, and the prevailing uncertainty. These concerns occupied my thoughts, creating a mental haze; however, I was ultimately aware that I must confront this challenge directly. The months preceding my surgery in February 2021 constituted an emotional tumult, characterized by episodes of anxiety, doubt, and frustration, as I questioned the propriety of my decision.

Despite these intense emotions, I maintained the hope that a more promising, seizure-free future was just around the corner. I reminded myself of numerous individuals who had embarked on a similar journey and emerged more resilient. I placed my confidence in my medical team, whose expertise and compassion provided reassurance, thereby helping me to feel more composed and prepared. On the day of the operation, I experienced a mixture of anxiety and resolve.

I recognized that brain surgery is among the most intricate and delicate procedures; however, I believed that miracles occur when proficient, skilled hands and compassionate hearts collaborate. The surgery marked a significant turning point. Although it was frightening, fraught with risks and uncertainties, I held onto the hope that it would signify a fresh start. And indeed, it was.

After surgery, everything changed. My seizures happened less often and were less severe. For the first time in years, I felt free, a joy that's hard to put into words. The uncertainty I'd faced was lifted, and I started living again, rather than just getting by. Recovery is a long, patient process, but the payoff has been worth every moment of uncertainty. My journey has taught me some valuable lessons: that resilience comes from being vulnerable, and true strength shines through when faced with adversity.

Learning to see epilepsy as just one part of who I am has been a game-changer. It's challenging, but it doesn't define me or make me less worthy. Instead, it's helped me develop qualities like patience, empathy, and a steady hope that keeps me moving forward. To anyone facing similar challenges, I want to remind you: You're stronger than you think. Your condition is a part of your life, but it doesn't control your future. With the right support, knowledge, and courage, you can overcome doubt and fear.

Every challenge is an opportunity for growth, and each setback serves as a springboard for a comeback. The healing journey is a winding path with obstacles, but every step forward shows your resilience. Remember, you're never alone in this. Reach out for support, learn more, and trust the process. The spark of hope is within you, waiting to ignite your healing and renewal. In the chapters to come, I'll share my entire experience, from preparing emotionally to the surgery and life after that. My goal is to guide you, offer comfort, and remind you that the impossible can become possible with faith, courage, and hope. Every recovery story starts with a single brave step, and I truly believe that.

Chapter 2:
Childhood and Early Life Memories

Growing Up with Epilepsy: A Life Shaped by Challenges and Courage

Living with epilepsy wasn't just a string of medical episodes for me; it was a deeply personal journey of growth, resilience, and self-discovery. As a kid, I felt like I was trapped in a world where my body would often betray me without warning, an unpredictable partner in a dance I never asked to join. I still clearly recall those moments when my limbs would shake uncontrollably, as if caught in a storm too fierce to handle.

My vision would blur, with colors merging into an indistinct haze, rendering my surroundings distant and surreal. The sense of helplessness that engulfed me upon realizing I could not halt the shaking was profoundly overwhelming, a frightening yet familiar sensation I wished to forget. During such episodes, I would be overcome by exhaustion as if struck by a formidable tidal wave. The physical repercussions of seizures extended beyond the convulsive episodes themselves. Subsequently, I would feel thoroughly depleted, as though I had completed an untrained marathon, with my body aching and my mind clouded.

It was an exhausting fatigue that lingered long after the seizures stopped, draining energy from every movement and filling my days with a weariness I couldn't shake off. Some episodes would drag on for several days, keeping me in bed, wrapped in blankets, as tremors still shook my limbs and my mind struggled with the haunting memory of what had happened. The pain during long seizures felt sharp and persistent like a dull ache that seemed to sink deep into my bones and muscles, a constant reminder of the invisible battle my body fought.

It's a quiet kind of warfare, fought in the shadows, where we often can't see the ongoing battles against fatigue, pain, and emotional struggles that we bear silently. Epilepsy isn't just about flashing lights or sudden convulsions that make headlines. It's a persistent, quiet presence that gradually overtakes your life, leaving you drained both physically and emotionally for days, weeks, or even months at a time.

I remember waking up, regaining consciousness, feeling confused, with a pounding headache that echoed the chaos in my mind. My limbs felt heavy and sore, like I'd just finished a tough workout, even though I hadn't moved much at all. Sometimes, I'd cry for reasons I couldn't fully understand, overwhelmed by the emotional weight of feeling disconnected from myself, my surroundings, and even from friends who couldn't fully understand what I was going through.

What was the hardest part? It was the isolation that came with feeling disconnected. I knew I was fighting something invisible that others couldn't see or understand. I recall lying in bed, shaking after a severe seizure, staring up at the ceiling as exhaustion set in. My body felt heavy and sluggish, and I was sometimes unresponsive. Even moving my arms was a struggle, and blinking took all my effort. My mind was fuzzy, and it felt like time had stopped. During these episodes, the outside world continued to move, but I was stuck in a silent storm within.

Going through these experiences, often alone and always in fear, was incredibly traumatic, not just for me but also for those around me, because they saw me struggle through the episode but couldn't help me more. Now, more than ever, I can only imagine the immense pain my family must have felt watching their child endure such intense suffering. The feeling of helplessness was almost overwhelming. Seeing a loved one in agony, watching their body tense up and their eyes cloud over, and knowing I had no control, just like them, is a memory that will always stay with me.

Over the years, I came to realize that epilepsy didn't just affect my body, it also changed who I was as a person. It forced me to face fears I never thought I'd have to confront about my safety, my future, and whether I could lead a normal life. But with every seizure and every bout of fatigue, I also found out that I was tougher than I thought. I was learning, often quietly, how to tune in to my body, how to ask for help when I needed it, and how to accept my limitations without losing hope.

There were occasions when I experienced feelings of defeat and fatigue from the relentless cycle of worry and recovery. However, I also encountered moments of discreet pride such as successfully navigating an entire day without a seizure or awakening after a prolonged episode with a glimmer of relief, acknowledging my survival through yet another storm. These minor achievements served as my anchors, reaffirming that I was more than my condition. They invigorated my determination to persevere and sustain hope, even when the future appeared uncertain or intimidating.

Growing up taught me priceless lessons about strength, those inner reserves that emerge strongest in times of adversity. It showed me the value of patience, humility, and empathy for others battling unseen struggles of their own. And it gave me a deep appreciation for the power of resilience, the ability to bounce back, even when the odds seem impossible.

My journey hasn't been easy, but it's made me who I am today: someone who knows the value of compassion, the power of perseverance, and the promise of hope. I'm sharing my story now because I know many others face similar struggles, silent warriors battling invisible battles. My hope is that my words remind you: no matter how tough the road gets, you're not alone. Your strength, like mine, comes from perseverance, courage, and the ability to keep moving forward, one day at a time.

The Family's Silent Battle

As a kid, I was completely caught up in my own struggles, the seizures, hospital visits, and endless medication, without realizing how much my epilepsy was affecting my family behind the scenes. Now, as an adult, I see how deeply they carried that invisible burden. My family, especially my parents, have always been my rock, even when I didn't notice their worries lurking beneath their calm exteriors. I remember those nights when I was sick, shaking through seizures, often unaware of how my body was betraying me.

They would stay close, with their eyes alert and tense, awaiting any signs that I was about to experience an episode. Their hands would tremble slightly as they gently supported me or endeavored to ensure my safety, even amid their efforts to maintain composure, a feat I now recognize required considerable strength. My mother, with her gentle yet firm voice, would softly reassure me, "You're okay," despite her own heart pounding with fear. My father, ever vigilant, became nearly instinctively attentive, learning to anticipate my seizures, discreetly shielding me from the prying eyes of neighbors and friends, and concealing his anxiety behind a mask of stoic resolve.

I can only imagine the helplessness they must have felt during those times. They might have been overwhelmed by tears, unconsciousness, or uncontrollable shuddering, and their sole actions were to wait, hope, and pray for each episode to pass safely. Witnessing their child's suffering and being limited to holding their hand or whispering reassurances was a silent struggle they endured daily, a burden they bore quietly, often in solitude.

Their constant vigilance touched every part of our lives. Parents, especially during my early years in the Dominican Republic, adjusted their routines, waking up early to prepare my medication, staying close during playtime, and always being prepared to respond at the first hint of trouble. It was draining, but they endured it with steadfast love and quiet strength.

Back in my childhood days, surrounded by the warm Caribbean sun, I was a carefree kid running barefoot on the soft, sandy shores of rivers, playing baseball with neighborhood friends, and feeling the wind in my hair as I sprinted through endless summer afternoons. The smell of ripe mangoes on the trees, the gentle lapping of waves on the shoreline, and the laughter of kids echoing under the vast blue sky were my moments of innocence, innocence I clung to tightly because I believed I'd one day live in a world free of fear and limits.

Those memories continue to evoke a gentle optimism within me, a hope that one day I will be able to breathe freely and run without fear. However, as I now reflect, I recognize that those carefree days were often interrupted by the shadows cast by my condition, fears that my seizures might recur, concerns about living up to my potential, and silent prayers for a future in which epilepsy would not confine me. My parents, especially my father, who lives in the Dominican Republic, where I grew up, were my guardians in every sense of the word: attentive, compassionate, and steadfast. They showed strength through silent acts of love, shielding me from chaos while bearing the full burden of anxiety and fear within their hearts.

Their unwavering care provided me with a sense of safety, even during times when I was unable to comprehend the danger I faced. Their concern manifested as a quiet, persistent whisper in the background of my childhood, an unspoken understanding that each seizure and episode represented a shared struggle they endured with the same determination as I faced my own.

Reflecting on these experiences, I now acknowledge that epilepsy has not only impacted my physical health but has also markedly influenced the dynamics of my entire family. It fostered enduring qualities such as resilience, compassion, and silent sacrifice. They assumed roles as caregivers, protectors, and occasionally, unspoken heroes bearing burdens that remain concealed from the external world yet are profoundly felt within their hearts. Throughout these challenges, I continue to carry their strength with me.

Their quiet strength, unwavering love, and sacrifices remind me every day that true courage isn't about being loud or proud; it's about the inner resolve we find during tough times, the unseen battles we fight with hope, faith, and unconditional love. My journey isn't just about me; it's a story of resilience, of a family that refused to give in to fear. And I share it because I want others to know that behind every quiet struggle, there's an unbreakable spirit. Even in the darkest moments, hope can still flourish, and healing can begin in the most unexpected places.

Living on the Sidelines

As I entered my teens, epilepsy started to feel like a wall that silently kept me apart from the world I desperately wanted to be a part of. I stood by and watched as others ran through the streets, jumped into rivers, or rode bikes with reckless abandon, all things I longed to do without hesitation.

I wished to submerge my toes in rivers, experience the wind rushing past my face during adventurous bicycle rides, and bask in the sun with a carefree smile. However, each time I envisioned engaging in these activities, my mind would be captivated by my father's cautious voice, his gentle cautions concerning the unpredictable nature of my body and the potential for seizures to occur without warning, transforming the moment into chaos.

He loved me intensely. His concerns came from a place of love, but they clouded my childhood, warning me to be cautious, to keep a low profile, to stay protected. I tried to suppress my envy of how I yearned to be like my friends, to laugh freely, to feel the freedom to move without fear. I admired their bravery, their ability to explore, and their genuine happiness.

My goal was to feel that pure, carefree happiness to be exhausted from running, beaming from triumph and heartbreak alike, not feeling stuck behind invisible walls that I couldn't rely on my own body to shatter. Yet, even in that yearning for freedom, I discovered small, precious sources of joy that became my sanctuary and identity.

When I felt like my body was out of control, sketching brought color and calm into my life, creating lines and shapes that helped me understand the chaos inside. I devoured books, stories of adventure, resilience, and hope, finding inspiration in the lives of others who had faced tough times and refused to give up. These creative pursuits became my sanctuary, a place where I could be myself, free from fear and limitations.

My teenage years were a blur of frustration and longing. I saw my friends sometimes diving into pools, others discovering new rivers, or racing through neighborhoods on scooters and bikes, living with a fearless joy I couldn't quite reach. They explored the world with confidence, their laughter filling the air, their energy endless. I desperately wanted to be like them to run, to jump, to feel the thrill of adrenaline, and not be held back by a secret enemy inside me.

There were many moments that felt like constant reminders of what I was missing. I envied their carefree attitude, the way they spoke up loudly, and how they embraced life's simple pleasures without hesitation. I watched as kids chased each other around, splashed water freely, and filled the streets with laughter and joy. Meanwhile, I sat quietly, often feeling like an outsider, observing a door I longed to walk through but was afraid to, out of fear of losing everything.

Despite feeling down and frustrated, I didn't let my situation completely crush my spirit. Instead, I found new ways to find happiness and meaning. I threw myself into music, investing my energy into my guitar and letting my songs express my hopes and fears. My sketches became a way to process my thoughts and give a voice to my emotions. Reading opened up new worlds for me, revealing stories of people overcoming adversity and finding hope, which I held onto when reality felt overwhelming. I also became involved in my community, participating in activities that made me feel connected, alive, and valued.

Whether it was volunteering, joining local youth groups, or simply sharing my story with others who understood my struggles, I learned that life can be rich and meaningful even when certain freedoms feel out of reach. Growing up with epilepsy during my teenage years made me a stronger and more empathetic person. It showed me that joy doesn't always come from running around or laughing loudly. Sometimes, it's found in quiet moments, the music that lifts your mood, the drawings that help you heal, or the friendships that understand your silence.

Although I still yearn to run free in the world, I've come to understand that my journey is about embracing what I've gained, not longing for what's missing. I've discovered resilience, creativity, patience, and a deeper appreciation for life's small, precious moments. While the shadows of my condition still linger, they no longer define me. I'm more than my limitations; I'm a person dedicated to living fully, with hope, courage, and the unwavering belief that even the deepest wounds can become sources of strength and inspiration.

Becoming a Source of Support for Others

Each day, I strive to be the kind of adult I once wished I had been, someone who meets others with kindness, patience, and full attention. I know from personal experience how lonely and overwhelming life can be, especially when facing challenges that others might dismiss or overlook. That's why I've made it my goal to be the person who listens more than

I talk, offers understanding before judgment, and truly cares about the well-being of those around me.

Teaching isn't just about passing on knowledge or offering guidance; it's about having faith in others that they're capable, valuable, and worthy of kindness, even when they can't see it themselves. When I show up with genuine confidence in my students, friends, or family, something special starts to happen; they begin to believe in themselves, too.

They recognize their strength and worth through my perspective, and that moment of validation often acts as the catalyst that motivates their continued efforts. You may have supported someone in the past, and now it's your chance to do the same for others. Life has shown us that small acts of kindness can make a significant difference. These could include a warm smile, a comforting word during a tough moment, or just being there without trying to fix everything. Even though these gestures might seem minor, they plant seeds of hope and trust that can grow into resilience and renewed confidence.

Every challenge I face on my personal journey, whether it involves managing my health, overcoming setbacks, or confronting my fears, reminds me that support is reciprocal. When I show compassion to others, I also gain strength in return. It's in moments of sharing, giving, and believing that deeper connections grow, leading to mutual growth. This reciprocal process embodies life's beauty: by supporting others, I find purpose; by receiving support, I find healing.

Consequently, I commit to demonstrating a consistent presence each day, being fully attentive and prepared to listen, recognizing that the presence of an individual who genuinely cares can have a profound impact. As I support others, I reaffirm my own hope that kindness and faith possess the capacity to heal wounds and inspire transformation. Ultimately, serving as a support for others pertains not only to those I assist but also to the ongoing development of my own character. Every act of kindness and belief I demonstrate stands as a testament to my personal growth, serving as a reminder that even amidst our individual struggles, we possess the ability to uplift others and generate ripples of hope that surpass our own challenges.

The Lessons Etched in Memory

Growing up with epilepsy in childhood taught me lessons most kids don't learn until much later—how to accept uncertainty, confront fear head-on, and find happiness despite life's persistent unfairness. I've come to understand that every person's journey is unique, with its own set of challenges and victories. Although my path included hurdles I didn't choose—unexpected seizures, hospital visits, and moments of helplessness—it also equipped me with invaluable life skills: resilience, empathy, and a profound gratitude for even the smallest wins. Epilepsy has been a part of my life for as long as I can remember. Some days, I've felt like I'm living on a fragile edge—knowing that my body's unpredictable nature could remind me of its presence at any moment. Yet, I've learned that this condition doesn't define me; instead, it influences my path without limiting it. It's a part of my story that has shaped my outlook, my strength, and my understanding of what truly matters. My experiences have shown me that when one dream is shattered—when I faced setbacks or fears—I discovered that new dreams could emerge—dreams more meaningful than the ones I initially envisioned. I once aspired to become a police officer, driven by a deep desire to serve my community, uphold justice, and protect those who couldn't protect themselves. I looked up to the heroes in law enforcement and the military—family members and mentors whose dedication and sacrifice inspired me. Their unwavering commitment to service fueled my own hope of making a difference, of creating positive change, and of making my neighborhood—and beyond—a safer place.

But as I learned more about my medical condition, I faced some tough realities. I had to confront the fact that certain aspects of my health might limit what I could do, or at least require me to approach my dreams with new caution. The risk of seizures during high-stakes situations, or the unpredictability of my health, made me question whether I could meet the demanding physical and mental standards of law enforcement. Those doubts were real—I felt frustration, disappointment, and a mixture of hope and fear. Yet, even in the face of those challenges, I refused to let my condition quietly diminish my aspirations. I began to see that limitations aren't final—rather, they are invitations to redefine what "service" and "strength" truly mean. Maybe my path wouldn't follow the traditional route, at least not exactly as I envisioned, but it could still be meaningful. I realized that my purpose—to serve, protect, and bring positive change—could take many forms. I could channel my passions into community advocacy, mentorship, or helping others navigate their own health journeys. Living with epilepsy has taught me patience—for myself and others. It's shown me that setbacks are part of progress, that hope can be persistent even when circumstances seem discouraging. Those lessons, learned early on in adversity, now serve as a foundation for every step I take forward. They remind me that resilience isn't about never falling but about how fiercely you stand back up. So, I embrace my story—its victories and struggles—as a testament to my growth. My journey has enriched me with empathy for those fighting unseen battles— be they health-related or emotional. And I carry within me the hope that, despite the obstacles, I can still make a difference—perhaps in a way I never initially envisioned, but one that still fulfills my desire to serve and protect.

Ultimately, I believe that adversity, when faced with courage and perseverance, can carve out a path toward a purpose more profound than we ever imagined. My story is still unfolding, and I am committed to forging a future rooted in hope, resilience, and service—ready to embrace the next chapter ahead.

A Path Redirected, Not Abandoned

When my medical evaluations showed that my epilepsy could be a major risk during intense physical training or high-stress situations typical in the tough world of law enforcement, it hit me hard. That reality, once it became clear, felt like an insurmountable obstacle, a barrier that seemed to make my goals even more out of reach. For a while, it stung deeply, as if a part of who I was had been put on hold or taken away altogether.

It's tough to face the fact that your dreams, so vivid and bold, might be limited by things you can't control. I felt a wave of disappointment and frustration, fighting the urge to see this as a sign of failure. The dream of joining law enforcement, of actively protecting and serving my community, suddenly seemed out of reach like a star I could no longer touch.

However, amidst that deep disappointment, I discovered a new source of strength and an understanding that sometimes life's plans can change and new opportunities can arise unexpectedly. I shifted my focus toward education, which felt equally vital to my purpose. I developed the aspiration to help others and to make a real, daily difference. I take pride in my role as a Paraprofessional within the New York City Public Schools system, officially known as the Department of Education of the City of New York, where I work with students in special education.

This profession has proven to be both enlightening and transformative. It requires significant qualities such as patience, creativity, and deep understanding. It is a calling that constantly demands adaptation to each student's individual needs, the development of innovative communication strategies, and the creation of a safe environment where students feel respected and understood. Working with children who face various challenges has greatly strengthened my belief in the importance of resilience. Each day, I witness moments of progress and small victories that underscore the importance of perseverance, compassion, and patience.

It is during these moments that I observe reflections of my personal journey confronting challenges, experiencing misunderstandings, and yet electing to advance with hope. This experience has demonstrated to me that limitations are not the end; rather, they serve as an encouragement to develop, acquire knowledge, and discover new approaches to serve. My past, characterized by struggles with epilepsy, no longer appears as an obstacle but rather as an essential part of my narrative that has cultivated my compassion and resilience. It is a chapter rich in lessons about hope, perseverance, and the ability to adapt.

My journey has demonstrated that, at times, true strength does not lie in adhering to the original plan but in possessing the courage to develop a new one that aligns with our genuine purpose. The unforeseen turns of life, rather than hindering us, can serve as catalysts for growth, compassion, and service. I firmly believe that our setbacks often serve as a prelude to new successes. Consequently, I continue to pursue this path with steadfastness, hope, and a dedication to making a meaningful difference in my own manner. My narrative is still evolving, and I eagerly anticipate what the future may bring, trusting that every experience, regardless of how challenging, enhances my resilience and capacity to uplift others.

The Most Profound Lesson I Have Learned

The most profound lesson I have learned is that our past does not define us, no matter how difficult, painful, or overwhelming those chapters might have been. My story with epilepsy is just one part of my journey. It's an important chapter, but not the whole story. I've realized that our true identity is shaped by how we respond to life's unavoidable challenges, whether they appear as health issues, setbacks, or unexpected changes, and by our ability to adapt and move forward with resilience and hope.

Having a condition like epilepsy meant dealing with moments of fear, frustration, and uncertainty. It often felt like I was carrying a heavy weight that I couldn't shake, a burden of things I couldn't control. There were times when I doubted everything: my worth, my future, my ability to succeed, and even whether I'd ever find peace. But during those tough times, I learned a crucial lesson that while I couldn't change what happened or the hand I was dealt, I could choose how I responded.

Every challenge transformed into an assessment of my resilience and adaptability. I was compelled to develop the ability to attentively listen to my body, identify warning signs, and advocate for myself in unprecedented ways. Even when overwhelmed by fear or fatigue, I persisted, sometimes gradually, sometimes with lingering doubts, but always with a determination to confront any circumstances with bravery. Instead of dwelling on limitations, I focused on what was within my control: my attitude, my effort, and my willingness to adapt to new situations.

Seeing things from this perspective completely changed my outlook. Life isn't about dodging hardships; it's about how we face them head-on. It's about building resilience as we learn to stand strong in the face of challenges and find meaning even in the midst of chaos. I came to understand that setbacks, though painful, are chances for growth, teaching us patience, humility, and inner strength. My own journey has taught me that our stories aren't fixed; they're dynamic, changing with each decision we make to adapt, learn, and stay hopeful.

Even in the toughest moments, when I was hurting or unsure, I realized that choosing to face life head-on and refusing to give up was what really defined me. I learned that resilience isn't about being unbreakable; it's about being willing to pick yourself up, rebuild, and grow stronger each time you're knocked down. Today, I realize that my past is just part of my story; it doesn't define my worth, abilities, or potential. What truly shapes us is how we respond when life throws us off track.

It is the courage to face new circumstances with an open heart, the humility to learn from setbacks, and the willingness to persist even when the road appears uncertain. This lesson continues to serve as a guiding principle, inspiring me daily to have confidence in my inner strength and to trust that, regardless of the challenges that may arise, I possess the ability to shape my future one decision at a time.

Chapter 3:
The Diagnosis: Confronting the Unknown

As I approached my surgery, my life seemed like a never-ending crescendo, a nonstop string of seizures that kept getting more frequent, intense, and unpredictable. Each episode felt like a warning, like my brain was saying, "I've reached my limit; I can't take this anymore." It was as if I could hear a distant alarm ringing, telling me my condition was getting out of hand, and that without help, I was headed for disaster.

Initially, the medications only provided temporary relief, like trying to cover a massive wound with fragile bandages. Doctors experimented with various drug combinations, each promising a breakthrough, but none lived up to my desperate hopes. Some pills left me feeling physically drained, with sore muscles and heavy limbs, as if I were already asleep. Others made me feel emotionally numb, disconnected from the world around me, as if I were watching life through a glass, unable to fully engage or experience the warmth of relationships.

Certain medications were excessively potent, clouding my cognition and causing me to forget simple words or moments of clarity, while others were too weak, leaving me exposed and vulnerable to seizures I couldn't predict. It felt like battling an unseen enemy that struck unexpectedly, much like a sudden storm catching me off guard in an open field. My seizures happened unpredictably, disrupting my daily routines and shattering my peace. Sometimes, I would be doing a task, and suddenly, everything would become blurry, my body would freeze, and my vision would turn dark.

I was powerless, entangled in a game with ever-changing rules, and each seizure appeared to diminish my sense of control and stability. The sound of time's passage grew increasingly loud in my mind, a constant reminder of my gradual detachment from the life I previously knew. I felt as if my body and, by extension, my very existence, were slowly unraveling. Every seizure left a lasting impact, not only physically scarred my brain and body, but also emotionally, eroding my hope and confidence. I would wake in the aftermath, disoriented, with a throbbing headache that mirrored the chaos within my mind.

My once-sharp focus and optimism had started to dwindle, giving way to a heavy cloud of uncertainty and helplessness. On days when seizures hit hard, I'd find myself retreating into a silent world. I'd lie there, drained, too exhausted to speak, too overwhelmed to fight. My thoughts would spin in circles, questioning and doubting, as I wished I could turn back time or wipe this invisible battle from my life. I felt like I was stuck in a storm that refused to let up, with no clear way out.

The experience was both humbling and often humiliating as I faced an unseen enemy that I couldn't understand or control, feeling as if I was gradually losing ground with each episode. There was a deep sense of fear, paired with profound loneliness. Days blurred into nights, and each day was a relentless fight for survival, both physically and emotionally. Sensory overload, panic, guilt, and frustration created a complicated web that was hard to untangle. When I looked in the mirror, I wondered who I was becoming and whether I would ever regain clarity or find peace.

The future seemed uncertain, unpredictable, and sometimes distressing. However, during those dark times, I held onto a faint hope that someday I might find a way to escape the chaos. Although the diagnosis was overwhelming, it represented a step toward understanding. It marked the start of a journey that forced me to face not only my medical condition but also the fears, doubts, and uncertainties that had become deeply rooted. I realized that confronting this head-on was the only way to move forward.

Medications That Failed to Provide Relief

At first, the medications I was taking seemed to bring some sense of control, but then they stopped working. I held onto hope that the new ones would help me feel better, maybe even reduce the number of seizures or how severe they were. But no matter how many combinations I tried, some stronger, some weaker, nothing really gave me the relief I was desperate for.

Instead, each new medication merely contributed to my frustration, inducing side effects that frequently exacerbated my feelings of exhaustion and helplessness. Each adjustment of dosage or change of medication resembled fighting a battle wherein the adversary continually altered its tactics. What initially appeared as a hope, a pill promising control, transformed into another obstacle, another instance of uncertainty. I observed increased fatigue in my body, with my energy depleting at an unprecedented rate.

My mind became increasingly foggy, impairing my ability to focus and remain present. The continuous challenges associated with my medication regimen left me in a perpetual state of fatigue, encompassing both physical and emotional dimensions, akin to running on empty in an unwelcome race. There existed a profoundly distressing sense that I was descending deeper into a tunnel with no apparent exit. Each setback exacerbated the impression that I was losing ground and that my condition was deteriorating rather than improving.

It felt like I was constantly battling an invisible force that kept shifting its tactics, making each day more difficult and uncertain. I often wondered, Will this ever improve? Or am I trapped in an endless cycle of trial and error? The frustration was amplified by the emotional toll of feeling imprisoned in my own body, exhausted from always adapting, and struggling with feelings of despair that sometimes surfaced during long, restless nights. I couldn't help but wonder if I was fighting a losing battle, caught in a war where I was exhausted but still holding on, refusing to give up.

But even in the darkest moments, I knew I had to keep moving forward to believe that somewhere, amid all this chaos, there was an answer, even if I couldn't see it yet. I had to hold on to hope, no matter how faint it seemed, remembering that sometimes, the greatest victories come after the hardest fights.

The Hospital Room: A Realm of Stark Reality

Being in the hospital room felt like being at home, a world that stayed the same, where each visit ran together. The sterile, white walls, the steady hum of machines, and the sound of wheels on the linoleum floors made a constant noise that almost drowned out my own thoughts. IV tubes dripped into my arm, their steady hum and the slight flicker of the monitor screens a constant reminder of being watched.

Wires were intricately woven across my body, connected to heart monitors, EEG caps, and other medical devices that monitored each heartbeat, brainwave, and movement. Their rhythmic beeping resembled a subdued heartbeat, occasionally comforting, at other times overwhelming, resonating with my feelings of solitude in a world where I perceived myself as merely another patient lost amidst a multitude of medical procedures.

Hours felt like an eternity as I lay confined to the hospital bed, my body fragile and weighed down, muscles stiff and sore from inactivity, limbs largely unresponsive and sluggish because I couldn't get out of bed until every test and procedure was over, while I stayed in the hospital. The sterile air pressed heavily around me, thick with antiseptic scents that seemed to seep into my skin, leaving a faint chemical sting behind. My mind often drifted into a fog, dazed from sleep deprivation, constant medications, and the overload of tests that left me feeling more like a puzzle piece rather than a whole person.

Each diagnostic procedure, whether it's a scan, MRI, EEG, or blood test, added more pieces to the complex puzzle of my health. However, instead of clarifying things, it only raised more questions. Was this progress? Did we truly understand the underlying issues? Will I ever find real peace? Lying there, exhausted, I would look up at the ceiling, lost in thought, weighed down by my circumstances. The white ceiling tiles blended into a uniform expanse as my mind grappled with the endless cycle I was caught in.

"Will this ever end?" I wondered. "Will I find a way out of these inner storms, these tidal waves of fear, pain, and exhaustion?" Those haunting questions echoed in my mind day and night, fueling an internal struggle from which I could not escape. Occasionally, I felt as if I were suffocating, overwhelmed by the burden of perpetual testing and treatment, the effort to regain mastery over my body and mind appeared unceasing, akin to engaging in a protracted conflict with no apparent conclusion.

Despite the physical discomfort, the emotional turmoil proved nearly as burdensome to endure. The white walls, unaltered routines, and the constant beeping and humming of machines became emblematic of my silent struggle, occasionally resembling a trap, a cage from which I felt unable to escape. Each new test or adjustment in medication elicited a mix of hope and anxiety, creating an unceasing cycle that rendered me increasingly exhausted with each passing day.

The silent ache of uncertainty gnawed at me: Am I ever going to feel normal again? However, amidst the chaos, a quiet, persistent voice remained deep inside. It refused to fade away, serving as my inner anchor amid the turmoil. This voice acted as a reminder, especially during my loneliest moments, that I was not fighting this struggle alone. I was not alone. I thought about the many others who had faced similar challenges and fought and endured.

Their stories were my quiet reminder that I wasn't alone. The way they faced the unknown with resilience showed me that this challenge wasn't mine to bear, that even in the darkest moments, there was still hope. That calm, unwavering voice became my steady ground, my silent partner. It whispered that even when everything seemed like an endless struggle, I had a strength within me that no machine or medication could measure, a resilience built on hope, faith, and a refusal to give up.

It made me realize I am more than just my tests, seizures, or fears. Even in the darkest moments, I have the strength to keep moving forward. So, with each passing day, I hold on to that inner voice, trusting that I can face whatever comes next, driven by the quiet confidence that I am resilient. This is an ongoing struggle, yes, but also a testament to my courage, perseverance, and unbreakable spirit.

Exploring the Path of Diagnostics: An Endless Journey

Those endless days are etched in my memory as a never-ending sequence of diagnostic tests that felt more like rituals than moments of healing. Each scan, MRI, EEG, and appointment was like a chapter in a complex story my body was trying to tell, but couldn't quite express. The sterile smell of antiseptic, the flickering overhead lights, and the coldness of the hospital bed became part of the routine. Whenever I was hooked up to wires and machines, the soft beeping filled the room, sometimes a calming rhythm, sometimes a relentless reminder of my ongoing struggle.

Days frequently blended into nights within that sterile environment. Hours extended interminably as I remained confined to a hospital bed, my body feeling more fragile than I had ever anticipated, unable to stand unassisted, trembling from exhaustion, and my muscles weakened by inactivity. The numerous tubes inserted into my veins conveyed medications I hoped would aid my recovery, yet they often contributed to the sensation of being trapped in an endless cycle of dependency. The soft hum of machines served as both a lullaby and an alarm, constant, steady, and all-pervasive.

The medical team moved quietly around me, showing seriousness along with compassion. They carefully reviewed my reports, took notes, and discussed my case with a quiet sense of urgency. Their conversations, full of scientific terms and complex theories about the brain's mysteries, often made me feel overwhelmed and helpless. The brain is an incredibly complex organ, surprisingly delicate yet remarkably resilient. At that moment, it felt as if my entire sense of self was wavering, fragile, and uncertain.

Each seizure left me feeling physically exhausted, like I'd been hit by a wave of fatigue I couldn't shake off. My muscles shook, my head throbbed with a dull pain, and a deep emotional vulnerability took over, leaving me feeling anxious and helpless. During one especially long hospital stay, my body shaking uncontrollably and my mind overwhelmed with pain and despair, I recall staring at the ceiling, trying to hold on to tiny bits of hope as the soft hum of the machines surrounded me. The sterile white walls, the faint smell of disinfectant, and the steady beeping were all I could focus on as I struggled under the heavy weight of my situation.

During those moments, I wondered if this ordeal would ever truly come to an end or lead to a better lifestyle. I questioned whether I would ever find relief from the internal turbulence that constantly swirls within my mind and body. This question haunted me, especially during sleepless nights filled with tears and relentless thoughts. I stayed there, feeling exhaustion seep into every fiber of my being, longing for a moment of peace, and praying for the chaos to stop, hoping to find balance amid the unending storm inside.

Those anxious nights often became quiet struggles, driven by fear of what might happen and uncertainty about whether I would ever find my way back to a life of freedom and happiness. Every new test, every appointment brought either hope or despair, but never a definitive answer. The journey felt like a puzzle with pieces scattered everywhere, leaving me feeling more vulnerable and more human. Living in that space of vulnerability taught me patience and resilience. I learned that healing isn't always a straight path; it's a slow, painful crawl through the dark.

Even with all the uncertainty, I held onto a small flicker of hope that this storm would eventually pass. That the struggle, though fierce, was also strengthening me, making me someone who could endure and overcome the chaos. Looking back now, I realize that those nights of pain and those days of trials, though exhausting, taught me lessons in endurance, patience, and hope. They're a reminder that even in the darkest moments, resilience can rise, and light can find its way back to the soul.

Reaching a Critical Moment: Considering Surgery

At that moment, a single word changed everything. When my neurologist mentioned the possibility of surgery, it felt as if time slowed down, and suddenly, the sterile atmosphere grew heavier, weighed down by unspoken fears and hopes. The word "surgery," often associated with fear, uncertainty, and the unknown, gained a new significance in that quiet conference room. It was a flicker of something new, something that could potentially alter the course of my life. I remember sitting up straight, my heart pounding so loudly I thought the neurologist could hear it.

My heart was racing with adrenaline, each beat pounding in my ears as my mind flooded with questions about surgery. Was that really an option for me? I had previously inquired about it, only to be told that it was not feasible, perhaps too risky, too complicated, or simply too uncertain for someone in my situation. That response had become a core part of my story, representing a barrier I saw as insurmountable. But when I heard it again, something shifted. I felt a deep change in my perspective, and the heavy cloud of doubt began to lift, replaced by a flicker of hope.

Our eyes locked, and I felt a surge of curiosity along with a faint spark of trust. Instinctively, I asked, "When can we begin? I am prepared." My voice carried a mix of excitement and determination that I hadn't felt in a long time. The doctor's polite smile and calming tone helped ease my growing anxiety. He gently tousled my hair and said, "Hold on, Roy. We need to do more tests first. Our goal is to make sure this is the right course of action for you. The most important step is to find the exact spot in your brain where the seizures start, the most delicate part of this procedure."

"Precision is everything; it's not just about the surgery, but doing it safely and effectively." His words carried weight, spoken with calm confidence, acknowledging that this wasn't a decision to be taken lightly. It marked the start of a long, carefully planned journey, a path that would span nearly two years and be filled with hope, anxiety, setbacks, and unwavering determination. As I listened, a mix of emotions washed over me. There was hope the possibility that this surgery could bring longer periods of freedom, free from the constant cycle of seizures and medications.

However, there was also an underlying fear, profound and visceral, concerning the delicate space within my mind where a mistake could entail more than mere disappointment; it could result in the loss of the limited control I believed I possessed. Even at that juncture, I was aware that there was no possibility of retreat. That moment represented a pivotal turning point, a conscious decision to confront the arduous journey of exploration and uncertainty directly. Consequently, I proceeded with resolve, sustained by a fragile yet resolute hope. Throughout this emotionally tumultuous period, I experienced a broad spectrum of emotions: hope, frustration, anxiety, and ultimately, determination.

Let me assure you that you're not alone in your struggles. Your fears and doubts are real, but they don't have to control your future. Your resilience demonstrates the incredible strength of the human mind to persevere, fight back, and grow. That one conversation, with its cautious optimism and careful planning, marked the start of a journey that challenged me in every way. It was a path that lasted nearly two years, filled with numerous tests, consultations, setbacks, and moments of quiet hope.

Each step held significance, recognizing that embracing uncertainty is a natural part of the journey. So, I moved forward, carrying the emotional aftermath of that day, fear, frustration, but also a faint hope that someday, this challenge could become a turning point, a fresh start guided by resilience and a firm belief that even in the unknown, we have the strength to endure and the ability to transform.

Two Years Defined by Uncertainty and Courage

Over the past two years, I've had to draw on my patience and resilience in ways I never thought possible. I've spent countless hours in the hospital, undergoing procedures that probed the intricacies of my brain. Some of these tests were incredibly invasive, like the one where they inserted electrodes deep into my skull to monitor my brain activity. Although these tests provided valuable information, they also brought a lot of pain and discomfort. Every time I had to lie still during a procedure with metal implants, loud equipment, or sedation, it drove home just how delicate and complex my body's internal systems are.

Those hospital days blended into a routine I both feared and relied on: antiseptic mornings, the rasp of linen against my skin, fluorescent lights that obscured the time of day, and the constant, subdued hum of machines that brought both comfort and unease. The tape holding the monitoring leads tugged at my hair when I removed it, and for days afterward, I felt as if small parts of myself stayed on those monitors: numb patches, phantom pressures, and the strange metallic taste left after anesthesia. Nights were the hardest. The ward would settle into a muffled silence, only to be broken by distant alarms, the squeak of trolleys, or the soft footsteps of a nurse.

Sleep was fragmented; I learned to count my breaths and place my hand on my chest until the world slowed enough to allow a brief rest. Pain was not always sharp or obvious. Sometimes, it appeared as a foggy headache that blurred my memory, a heaviness behind the eyes, and nausea that made the world seem tilted. At other times, it was electric and unpredictable, reminding me that my brain was still adjusting to the change. Activities I once took for granted, such as stirring a cup of tea, recalling a friend's name, and going down a flight of stairs without holding the banister, became milestones I faced with humility. There were days when even simple conversations felt like climbing a mountain.

Words would linger just out of reach, and even the simplest topics required intense focus. Those losses were small in terms of medical risk, but huge in the daily struggle for dignity and respect. The emotional toll added up in subtle ways. I grieved for versions of myself I hadn't realized I'd lost: carefree mornings, a job I could do without mental exhaustion, and the spontaneous laughter that vanished before brain fog made me wary. There was also guilt: for missed birthdays, canceled plans, and times when my spouse had to take on more than we'd anticipated. At my lowest points, I felt ashamed of needing help, as if relying on others were a personal failing.

Nonetheless, during those delicate hours, I perceived a new source of courage: the unwavering support of a sibling who read to me for an hour when my concentration waned; the friend who acquired the skill to drive me to appointments and remained in the waiting room, sharing a quiet companionship; and the nurse who sat with me following a panic attack, instructing me to count the tiles on the ceiling until my pulse decelerated.

Rehabilitation pushed me to the edge of my patience. But physical therapists would celebrate even the smallest progress, like taking my first step without help or climbing stairs without getting winded, and those wins felt like a burst of sunlight. I know some of you may be wondering why physical therapy; remember, after brain surgery, you might feel a little confused, out of balance, but it's part of the process. Occupational therapy helped me relearn the basics of daily life, such as buttoning a shirt, making toast without burning it, and writing clearly enough to leave a note that made sense. Cognitive exercises seemed both ordinary and incredible at the same time: memorizing flashcards, practicing memory drills, and having conversations in the mirror.

My progress wasn't a straight line. I took two steps forward and one step back, and some setbacks lasted weeks. But each small victory accumulated, like pebbles forming a path I could walk on again. I also had to handle practical challenges, such as filling out insurance forms that required proof, discussing my capabilities with employers, learning how to ask for help without compromising my dignity, and spending nights reviewing medical bills while trying to hold onto hope. Those frustrations were everyday and overwhelming, and they showed me that resilience isn't just about being brave; it's also about managing paperwork, logistics, and quiet negotiations with institutions that decide how care is provided.

My coping strategies naturally fell into place. I started keeping a small notebook by my bed, not to track my symptoms but to jot down tiny moments of happiness: the way sunlight spread across the kitchen table, a sentence that made sense, or a visitor's laugh. Breathing exercises, short walks around the block, and setting small goals helped me get through tough times. I learned to ask for help in specific ways, like "Can you fold these shirts?" or "Will you come with me to this appointment?" which was easier for people to say yes to than a general "help me." Humor was also a lifesaver; laughing at silly hospital gowns and my own clumsy attempts to be normal brought some light to dark days.

What I learned most of all was how to live with uncertainty without letting it dictate every moment. Uncertainty shifted from being a looming cliff to a field I had to navigate sometimes without sight, sometimes with a companion, and sometimes by feeling my way step by step. I found that courage wasn't about not being afraid; it was about putting one foot in front of the other, even when the path was unclear. This journey transformed my priorities and made me more grateful for what I have.

Since then, I've started noticing kindnesses I might have missed before: a janitor who always remembers my name, a neighbor who brings over soup, and a volunteer who brings a crossword puzzle to fill a dull afternoon. Two years later, my life is still different from what it was before surgery. That's both a painful reality and a precious gift. I'm more cautious and more understanding, more likely to appreciate small wins and sit with uncomfortable feelings instead of rushing past them.

The future remains uncertain; however, it is also marked by routines and rituals that bring stability: morning stretches that ease tension in the neck, a weekly phone call with my sister that always ends with laughter, and a notebook that now records not only symptoms but also plans for a picnic, a short trip, and a possible book to write. If there's one sincere lesson to share, it is this: courage is built through daily acts of perseverance and release.

When control over every aspect isn't possible, you still have the power to decide how to face each day. Stay curious about your resilience, be confident in asking for support, and believe that small, steady steps add up to a life rebuild.

"You have power over your mind, not outside events. Realize this, and you will find strength." — Marcus Aurelius

The Hidden Power of the Mind

The mind, I realized, is remarkably powerful. It can serve as either a source of strength or a constraining force. When the body is weakened, our minds have the capacity to elevate us or to restrain us. It can facilitate healing or induce suffering. Following my surgical procedure, I was required to learn how to communicate with myself differently, how to transform fear into motivation, and pain into purpose. Initially, it resembled the challenge of calming a storm. Evenings were filled with replayed worst-case scenarios: the failure of the surgery, persistent memory loss, and a life confined to appointments and medication.

In the darkness, my thoughts transformed into a distinct form of pain, rapid, intense, and elusive. I would remain awake, listening to my heartbeat, and contemplating statements such as, "I'll never improve," "This is too much," or "I'm weak." These thoughts acted as attractors, drawing me toward a state of panic. The initial step toward regaining control involved recognizing these thoughts before they overwhelmed me. I learned to articulate them aloud: "There's the worry voice," I would say quietly in the ward. Through this act of naming, they were removed from my mind and placed on the floor, where they appeared less threatening.

Managing my inner dialogue wasn't about denying my fears; it was about acknowledging them. It was about training my mind, just like a muscle. Sometimes I did that with deliberate practice, and other times it happened by chance, a habit that formed because it actually worked. I started carrying a small notecard in my pocket labeled "When Fear

Visits." On it, I wrote down brief, helpful responses I could remind myself of: "This is tough, not impossible," "What's one small step I can take right now?" and "I've gotten through tough times before."

Whenever I caught myself thinking, "I'll never get better," I'd gently push back. What proof do I have? Two months ago, I could only last five minutes; now I can walk down the block. Progress is real, even if it's not huge. Using practical strategies helped me stay grounded. When my head started spinning with worst-case scenarios, I'd use techniques to bring myself back to the present. I'd do the 5-4-3-2-1 exercise (focusing on five things I see, four things I feel, three things I hear, two things I smell, and one thing I taste) or hold a smooth river stone and describe its weight and texture until my breathing slowed down.

What I discovered was that I could schedule worry like a meeting, setting aside ten minutes in the late afternoon to work through my fears, then closing the book until the next day. This wasn't about denying my worries; it was about managing them, keeping them from consuming every minute of my life.

Cognitive reframing was another technique I employed. Whenever I thought, "I'm weak," I trained myself to rephrase it as: "I am recovering." When overwhelmed by pain, I asked myself: "What does this pain mean right now? What actions can I take?" Breaking down large, intimidating statements into smaller, manageable tasks, such as drinking water, calling my nurse, or resting for twenty minutes, helped turn panic into a problem-solving mindset. This approach kept me from becoming overwhelmed by emotions and gave me a sense of control, even if only a little. Therapy and structured rehab played a key role in this process.

A neuropsychologist instructed me on maintaining thought records, which include identifying the trigger, the automatic thought, evaluating the evidence for and against it, and considering a balanced alternative. Over time, patterns became evident, as specific triggers consistently elicited the same spirals, and recognizing these patterns enabled me to intervene effectively. Participation in group therapy and a small online support community was also beneficial; listening to others' candid admissions, such as "today I yelled at my spouse because I was scared," reduced my shame regarding my own complex inner experiences.

There were also small, ritualistic practices that carried great emotional weight. Before a tough appointment, I'd take three deep breaths while repeating to myself that everything would be okay, I was strong, and life was beautiful. During long periods of inactivity, I'd close my eyes and visualize walking along a familiar path, exaggerating the sensory details until my brain felt like it had rehearsed the movement. I wrote inspiring mantras on sticky notes, such as "I can do hard things," and stuck them on my bathroom mirror. On bad days, I'd reread a short list of three real accomplishments from the week, such as calling a friend, taking a ten-minute walk, or making a healthy meal, so I could focus on the small wins.

Control wasn't straightforward. There were days when a single sentence, someone's worried expression, or a bad test result would send me spiraling back into old patterns. That was part of the process: learning to be kind to myself when my mind defaulted to fear. Shame and self-criticism only reinforced the negative cycle. Instead, I learned to say, "That thought makes sense right now," and then shift my focus. Recovery required patience, including repeated practice, compassion, and the willingness to try techniques over and over until they became automatic responses.

The power of the mind also manifested in purpose. Pain that once appeared insignificant transformed into a valuable teacher. I commenced journaling not only symptoms but also insights gained about myself each week, an unanticipated smile, an act of bravery, a new boundary I established. These entries progressively restructured my narrative from "victim of circumstance" to "active participant in recovery." I found purpose in minor actions: replying to a single email, assisting another patient in sharing their story, and instructing my sibling on how to prepare my favorite soup. Such choices reinforced a self-image that was proactive rather than passive.

If there's one practical takeaway I want to highlight, it's this: While you can't always control what happens to your body, you can build habits that shape your mental reactions. Start small: notice your thoughts, keep a journal of a single small achievement each day, learn one grounding technique, and create a compassionate counter-statement to use during moments of distress. Strength doesn't mean the absence of vulnerability; instead, it involves recognizing your vulnerabilities and choosing to keep going anyway. True strength is found in everyday, repetitive acts, such as choosing a kinder thought, taking a deliberate breath, and consistently practicing until these choices become your mind's new default.

The Brain's Hidden Puzzle: The Origin of My Seizures

After months or even years of testing and consultation, my medical team identified the seizures as originating from my right temporal lobe, the region located just above the ear that plays a vital role in integrating memory, emotion, and self-awareness. The MRI images were both clinically informative and strangely personal: a high-resolution scan revealed hippocampal sclerosis, a subtle yet unmistakable scarring and volume loss in the hippocampus, a small curved structure essential for the formation of new memories. On the radiologist's screen, the affected hippocampus appeared shrunken compared to the contralateral side; on the T2/FLAIR sequences, a faint hyperintensity indicated residual injury.

The phrasing "sclerosis" and "chronic change" felt sterile within the meeting room; however, I comprehended the implication: this was not an instantaneous issue. It possessed a history. The remainder of the diagnostic puzzle cohesively aligned in a manner that was simultaneously reassuring and alarming. Extended video-EEG monitoring documented multiple clinical seizures, with the electrical onset consistently originating from the right temporal electrodes. This observation was consistent with the findings suggested by the imaging.

A PET scan revealed a small region of hypometabolism in the same area, confirming that the tissue was comparatively less active than expected. My team elucidated the limitations inherent in each diagnostic modality, the potential for scalp EEGs to obscure clarity, and the necessity of correlating clinical signs with imaging findings, yet the convergence of MRI, PET, and video-EEG robustly supported the diagnosis.

Looking back at the seizure, I noticed how the semiology correlated with the location. My auras, those early, strange moments before a full seizure, were small and vivid: a sudden, intense wave of déjà vu, a fizzy sensation in my chest, or an odd phantom smell that no one else could notice. During these events, I'd stare blankly, my hands would fumble at invisible clothes, and sometimes I'd make lip-smacking movements.

Afterward, I'd struggle to get my bearings, feeling confused and drained for minutes or hours. Those postictal gaps explained why I'd miss conversations and exits, and why there were holes in my memory from certain days. The right temporal focus also helped make sense of the emotional ups and downs. I later learned from my therapist that the mood swings and sudden outbursts of grief or fear were due to disruptions in the circuits that control emotions.

When the doctors told me that the scarring was "likely caused by a long-standing condition," the word "likely" carried a lot of weight. They looked into common causes: a history of prolonged febrile seizures during childhood, an old head injury that I might not remember clearly, or a past infectious or inflammatory event that made the hippocampus vulnerable. For many people with hippocampal sclerosis, the scarring is the result of a process that started many years earlier.

For me, it was like doing detective work in reverse, asking my parents about childhood fevers, digging through old records, and trying to link up a dot I hadn't even realized was there. The team didn't push me toward a single answer. We held multidisciplinary meetings with neurologists, epileptologists, neuroradiologists, and a neurosurgeon, who reviewed the images and seizure recordings together.

We discussed realistic outcomes and potential risks. Surgical options, such as an anterior temporal lobectomy or a more targeted amygdalohippocampectomy, were mentioned as possibilities that could significantly reduce or even eliminate seizures in many patients with hippocampal sclerosis. However, the discussion remained cautious: the hippocampus plays a vital role in memory, and removing or altering tissue there carries a real risk of affecting certain types of recall or emotional processing.

Through language and memory lateralization assessments, including functional magnetic resonance imaging (fMRI) and Wada testing in certain cases, we aimed to evaluate the potential effects of surgery on my daily memory function. Beyond clinical consultations, the diagnosis significantly changed practical aspects of my everyday life. Driving was restricted until seizure control was achieved; additionally, I learned to ask for help with cooking and stair navigation on days when my memory was impaired.

Medications temporarily decreased the frequency of symptoms; however, they were accompanied by side effects such as fatigue, cognitive clouding, and episodic mood fluctuations. These issues underscored the close interconnection between my treatment and my personal identity. Additionally, there were logistical challenges, including preauthorization procedures, scheduling supplementary neuropsychological assessments, and coordinating time off work for monitoring admissions.

Emotionally, getting the diagnosis was a strange kind of relief. I finally had a name and a place for the chaos, but it also brought a lot of sadness for the lost memories and the uncertainty about what life would be like after treatment. In quiet moments, I'd revisit the scans on my flash drive and look at that small, scarred hippocampus with a mix of anger and compassion. It reminded me that my seizures weren't a moral failing or some random, cruel thing; they were the result of a long process in a very small, vital part of my brain.

Understanding the origin did not eliminate fear; rather, it provided me with a strategic framework: conducting targeted testing, meticulously assessing risks and benefits, and formulating a plan grounded not solely in hope but supported by converging clinical evidence. This clarity, clinical, technical, and profoundly personal, served as the foundation for the decisions I was required to make regarding treatment, safety, and the reconstruction of the aspects of my life that seizures had disrupted.

Chapter 4:
The Day of the Surgery

That morning felt different in a way I couldn't quite put my finger on. I woke up around 4:00 a.m., feeling calm and without any panic; instead, I felt a quiet readiness that was almost spiritual. The hours leading up to surgery were filled with small, purposeful moments that helped me feel centered. In the pre-op area, the nurses moved with smooth efficiency. I changed into a hospital gown that smelled faintly of detergent, and they gently wrapped a thin blanket around my shoulders.

They placed a notecard with my name and birthdate on the hospital chart. The doctors applied a small numbing spray and then inserted an IV. A brief sting followed by the calming feeling of saline flowing. Standard checks were performed: name, procedure, allergies, and signed and initialed consent forms. The surgeon stopped by, sat on the edge of the bed, and explained everything calmly and clearly; his reassurance eased the trembling that often lingered beneath my composure. Family members arrived while it was still dark.

We exchanged the small courtesies that support important decisions: a long handshake, a whispered joke, and a final prayer shared together. I remember the corridor lights flickering from the fluorescent hum to the bright white of the operating room door. The movements were deliberate, the wheels squeaked, and my heart beat in rhythm with that motion.

Inside the OR, the space seemed bigger and quieter than I'd expected: high, clean lights, rows of monitors, neatly arranged trays of instruments, and a team that moved in perfect sync. The anesthesiologist introduced himself and walked me through the plan, using the same calm, clear voice surgeons use, making time for questions. He gently placed the oxygen mask over my face for a quick breath test; the mask had a faint, plastic-like, and antiseptic smell, and the oxygen tasted like a cool breath on my tongue.

He told me they'd also give me a small dose of sedative to calm my nerves before the more powerful anesthetic. There was a moment that felt both ceremonial and deeply human: everyone paused to do the surgical "time-out", verifying my name, the procedure, and the site. The nurse used a marker to ensure they had the correct temple; the surgeon's hand hovered over the area, as if blessing the spot where the operation would take place. A circulating nurse gently held my hand for a few seconds. In that brief touch, I felt reassured and understood that I wasn't just being checked off a list, but that I was being acknowledged as a person.

They sterilized my scalp with a strong antiseptic. The sharp, slightly bitter smell of chlorhexidine filled the air, and small pieces of gauze were tucked under my head to protect my hair. Sterile drapes created a private space around my face and shoulders, making the rest of the room a blurry background of light and movement. I heard the soft hum of the ventilators starting up, the clicks of the anesthesia machine, and the distant sound of surgical instruments being arranged.

A warming blanket was gently placed over my legs; the warmth eased the clinical coldness. Before the final induction, the anesthesiologist stayed by my head, repeating the names and doses of the medications to be given and reassuring me of continuous monitoring. I felt no sense of abandonment, only focused attention, as if everyone shared a common goal. I quietly said a brief prayer, mainly expressing gratitude rather than making a plea, and I sincerely thanked the team aloud.

The commencement of anesthesia was progressive, a warm influx emanating from my arm and extending through my chest. Initially, I experienced a sensation of heaviness, followed by a gentle spinning, akin to being enveloped in a soft fog. I noticed that my eyelids were becoming increasingly heavy. The overhead lights appeared to sharpen, then fade; the monitor beeps elongated into a lullaby. This experience was not intimidating. It resembled stepping off a familiar precipice into something simultaneously unfamiliar and reassuring.

Even as I drifted into unconsciousness, a sense of gratitude lingered like a steady, odd thread that carried me through the morning. I was thankful for the skilled surgeons' hands, the nurses who had held my hand, the prayers that gave me strength, and for the fragile, fierce hope that this was a new beginning rather than an ending. I came to later in recovery, surrounded by bright, muffled voices and the slow, measured footsteps of people moving just out of my awareness.

My mouth was dry, my throat sore from the breathing tube, and a soft pillow cradled my head. The surgeon stopped by with a few quiet words about how things had gone; I was too foggy for details, but I heard the words "procedure as planned" and felt a sudden, physical relief wash over me. Pain and confusion would come later, of course, but in that first tough and vivid afternoon, the memory that stuck with me was of hands that squeezed, hands that reassured, the steady hands of the team that had guided me through the most uncertain part of my journey.

As I whispered, "Thank you for helping me on my path to a better life. Thank you for guiding me through this process," I felt like I was regaining some control in a situation where everything seemed out of my hands. The inner light inside me seemed to shine brighter than the fear that surrounded me: faith, gratitude, and a steady conviction that I wasn't alone. Even as machines blinked and staff moved with precision, the room felt enveloped in something bigger: love, hope, and a higher power. The surgery itself took about eight to nine hours.

My memories of the OR are of a cool, sterile environment, the gentle hum of machinery, and the calm, competent atmosphere surrounding me as the team worked. As I drifted off, my last conscious thoughts were prayers and affirmations, short, steady mantras that felt like anchors. Then my body remained still for nearly nine hours, while my spirit seemed to float on a thread of trust. When I finally came to, I was in the ICU, still foggy from the anesthesia. My throat was sore from the breathing tube, my mouth tasted metallic, and a persistent, dull nausea lingered just beneath the surface.

The lighting appeared somewhat overly intense, and the sounds of the nurses' footsteps seemed muffled; however, through the haze, one face came into clear focus: my father. He had traveled from the Dominican Republic and was present, his eyes encircled with a mix of exhaustion and affection. Observing him at that moment, lean, fatigued, and somehow remarkably composed, felt akin to a benediction. He seated himself nearby, his hand warm in mine, murmuring prayers in Spanish that I could only partially perceive but which provided profound comfort. The rhythm of his voice held greater significance than the exact words spoken.

ICU life had its own rhythm. The room was filled with a gentle hum of soft beeps, infusion pumps, heart-monitor alarms, and the muffled sound of oxygen. An oxygen cannula sat under my nose, and thin lines connected me to IV poles carrying fluids, pain medication, and antibiotics. A clear dressing covered the shaved patch of scalp, and I could feel slight tension and a faint bruise where the surgeons had worked. Later, the surgeon pointed out a neat incision line along my temple, partially hidden by gauze and a small drainage tube; seeing it made the whole experience feel more real. Nurses performed frequent neurological checks: "Squeeze my fingers," "Follow my finger," "Can you stick out your tongue?" quick, practical tests that felt less clinical and more personal, as if they were checking for the return of the person I knew.

Pain came in waves, some sharp, some like a heavy pressure behind my eyes. The team managed it carefully—IV analgesics that took the edge off, anti-nausea medication, and regular comfort checks. I remember being taught how to cough and breathe into a small plastic device—the incentive spirometer—blowing until the gauge moved, a simple exercise meant to keep my lungs clear. It seemed trivial and heroic at once: each breath was a small reclaiming of my body. There were moments of disorientation. For a while, I wasn't sure of the day or exactly where I was; time had smeared. Family members became anchors.

When the surgeon arrived for rounds, I finally felt a genuine sense of relief wash over me. He spoke in a gentle tone, giving me a brief, calm update: "Everything went as planned," "no complications," "we'll keep an eye on the swelling." Those words hit me like a solid foundation after a long stretch of uncertainty. The care team then reviewed the next steps, which included close monitoring, imaging to track swelling, and a plan for gradually increasing mobility and physical therapy. Having a clear, manageable, and hopeful plan helped ease my anxiety.

Small routines began to piece the day together. A nurse brought me ice chips and a damp towel for my forehead; another helped me sit up on the edge of the bed for the first time, my legs wobbly but determined.

Each small milestone, sitting up, eating a full meal without feeling nauseous, recalling a child's name, felt like a step toward reclaiming my life. I also had to face the vulnerability of needing help with simple tasks, such as using the restroom, taking a shower, and getting dressed. That humbling dependence was tough, but it was also where I felt the most genuine kindness: the way a nurse gently smoothed my hair, the way my father joked to coax a smile out of me, the surgeon's calm reassurance.

As the day gave way to night, I felt drained and vulnerable, yet also lifted by a sense of gratitude. The pain and bandages were proof of the progress made, and each beep of the monitor seemed less ominous and more like a reassuring pulse keeping pace with my recovery. I whispered my thanks, quiet prayers of gratitude and promise, trusting that every breath and every small step were part of a larger healing process.

After the surgery, they wheeled me into the Intensive Care Unit and the world condensed into a handful of urgent, intimate details: the steady beeping of monitors, the soft hiss of oxygen, the cool tug of sheets against my skin. Anesthesia left me woozy and nauseated; my mouth tasted metallic, and every blink felt like lifting a curtain. My vision swam, but through the haze a shape resolved into something steady and beloved, my father.

My mother was also present, providing a constant source of warmth by my side. Her hands, cool yet confident, gently smoothed the blanket on my lap and offered soft words of encouragement, familiar refrains she had employed throughout my entire life. She advised me to sip water slowly, to consume small bites once the nausea subsided, and to practice the breathing exercises demonstrated by the nursing staff. Her voice served as a comforting balm: pragmatic, familiar, and consistently affectionate. When my perception of time or the sequence of events became unclear, she would succinctly recount the details in short, simple sentences until my scattered thoughts were reoriented.

A small collection of visitors' cards, a bouquet from colleagues, and a playlist curated for me, these tokens imbued the sterile environment with a sense of humanity. I was deeply moved by the outpouring of support that went beyond my immediate family: coworkers who adjusted their schedules to visit during designated hours, a supervisor who provided daily updates to my team to help with ongoing projects, and friends who maintained a continuous thread of messages and prayers within a group chat.

Those messages arrived at the most unusual hours, small bubbles of light on my phone that seemed like lifelines. Even the simplest messages, such as "Thinking of you" or "We're here when you're ready," carried significant weight. Volunteers and the hospital chaplain also visited, offering silent prayers or a listening ear. Their presence served as a reminder that recovery extends beyond the physical; it is intrinsically connected with community support.

Emotionally, the experience encompassed a combination of gratitude and vulnerability. I experienced joy from the presence of my parents, guilt regarding their concern, and profound appreciation for the fundamental human connection they offered. I subsequently came to a renewed understanding that pivotal moments are not isolated incidents; rather, they are sustained by the support extended by others. This insight fundamentally altered my perception of strength.

My strength came not just from enduring the surgery, but also from accepting and embracing the love and practical support I received, allowing others to take on what I couldn't do for a time. That memory, my father's silhouette lit by the ICU light, my mother's fingers tracing patterns on the blanket, the chorus of supportive messages still stays with me. It showed me that gratitude isn't just a feeling, but an action: thanking people, letting them see the impact of their help, and remembering to pass that kindness on when I can.

The early hours after surgery revealed a fundamental truth: humans are naturally made for connection, and being present during crises is one of life's greatest blessings. The gathering of family and friends around me not only showed their love but also uncovered a deep well of inner strength I hadn't fully realized within myself strength that would carry me through the tougher days ahead.

A Fight for Freedom

My battle wasn't with an outward enemy, but with an inner one, seizures that had been secretly running my life for too long. This procedure felt like a declaration of defiance, a public and private statement that I believed in living beyond those limitations. Lying on the operating table, I wasn't a passive observer; I was a warrior in silence, facing fear with every bit of courage I'd developed over the years. The sensory details are still vivid.

The oxygen mask rested coolly and slightly damp against my upper lip; the elastic strap emitted a soft hum as it settled behind my ears. The room was filled with the scent of antiseptic and polished metal, a sharp, clinical aroma that unexpectedly mingled with the subtle sweetness of hand lotion applied by a nurse. Overhead lights illuminated the space with an intensity comparable to that of the sun, and the voices of the surgical team were calm and precise, marked by brief exchanges of names, instruments, and confirmations.

For a brief moment, everything outside my body faded into the background; inside, I focused on the rhythm of the slow inhale, the long exhale, the steady beat of my own heart. I whispered affirmations to myself as if they were protective charms: You are safe. You are strong. You are entering a healing phase. Waking up in recovery was its own kind of battle: a mix of sensations I had to navigate like a minefield.

My scalp was tight and numb along the incision, and when the nurse carefully removed a corner of the dressing, I experienced a sudden, intense realization: there it was, the physical evidence of the confrontation. The bandage concealed precise stitches and a small drainage tube; the surgeon subsequently described it as "as tidy as we could hope for." These words resonated with a sense of achievement.

Recovery demanded patience and small acts of bravery. The first twenty-four hours were a mosaic of checks and minor victories: nurses gently encouraged me to breathe deeply with the incentive spirometer, helped me sit up at the edge of the bed for the first time, and monitored my grip strength and pupil response. Each neurological exam, including squeezing my hand, tracking my finger, and naming the month, felt both personal and intimidating, yet became somewhat reassuring once the responses were received. Pain came in waves; IV painkillers eased the worst discomfort, and I quickly realized the importance of asking for medication before a surge began.

That straightforward approach showed me how to be an advocate, even when I was at my most vulnerable. There were moments that were humbling. I needed help with the simplest things, using the restroom, getting dressed, and dealing with the dizziness that came with turning my head. But there were also moments that were quietly uplifting: my father's hand finding mine in the dim ICU light, my mother humming a lullaby that touched the parts of me that medicine couldn't reach, or a colleague's funny story that made me burst out laughing and forget my pain for a moment.

Visitors' cards, text messages, and a small bouquet from colleagues infused a sense of human warmth into the sterile hours. Each greeting of "How are you feeling?" conveyed greater significance than before. Sleep was fragmented; I drifted in and out of dozing, the morphine fog softening the edges of consciousness and the beeping monitors punctuating my dreams. Nighttime brought vivid, occasionally unsettling dreams, snapshots of my life interwoven with flashes of medical imagery.

As I woke from those dreams, I used the grounding techniques I'd practiced: I felt the weight of the sheet on my legs, named three things I could see in the room, and took slow, deliberate breaths until the world around me settled. Over the next few days, I gradually regained my footing. Physical therapists helped me stand up and take my first shaky steps; my legs trembled, but they held. Occupational therapists worked with me on fine motor tasks, such as buttoning a shirt and writing legibly enough to sign my name. A neuropsychologist assessed my memory and attention, not to judge me, but to understand the impact of the seizures and what could be rebuilt. Those sessions revealed both my strengths and weaknesses, and provided us with a plan – a truth that was both raw and encouraging.

There were setbacks that felt like punishment. One morning, a sudden spike in blood pressure delayed my discharge. Headaches would flare up unexpectedly with changes in the weather. I was constantly tired, and even simple conversations could leave me exhausted for the rest of the day. Each setback meant I had to adjust, get more rest, drink more water, and move at a slower pace. I learned to see setbacks as speed bumps, not cliffs. Medication became a constant companion, antiseizure meds that softened some of the rough edges in my thinking, but kept my seizures under control.

My neurologist and I worked together to find a balance between managing my seizures and staying clear-headed. We adjusted my medication, watched for side effects, and scheduled regular follow-up tests like EEGs and MRIs. Those appointments mixed feelings of anxiety and hope, as we gathered evidence that I could live a life less controlled by seizures. When the next EEG showed no immediate signs of seizures, I experienced a cautious optimism that was almost overwhelming. Small victories gave me a sense of freedom: my first full night's sleep without interruption, a week without a seizure, and the day I made coffee without accidentally turning on the stove.

Small celebrations became milestones for me, like taking a walk in the sunlight and feeling weightless, or going on a short drive with my doctor's okay, or laughing at a joke and remembering every word. Each victory reminded me that I was reclaiming parts of my life that fear had once taken from me. The spiritual and mental battles continued. Faith and fear coexisted within me; I learned to let faith guide me without ignoring the presence of fear. I relied on techniques like breathwork, prayer, and visualization, imagining my brain as a garden being nurtured, with roots growing stronger and new shoots emerging.

On tough days, I relied on mantras and small rituals that grounded me. I would place my hand over my heart and say a quick thank-you, close my eyes, and recall a memory of my parents' laughter, or recite the same psalm my father mouthed in the ICU. Over time, the scar faded into something more ordinary. Through rough patches and softer ones, the numbness around the incision slowly subsided in a jagged pattern. A small, raised line remained—a private reminder of a fight I had chosen.

My clinic visits included imaging, outpatient rehab, and discussions about weaning off medications if I remained seizure-free. Each checkup was an opportunity to assess my progress and reaffirm the decision I made in the OR that morning: to fight for my freedom. If I could pass on one truth to you, it's this: courage isn't about not being afraid; it's about taking a deliberate step forward despite fear.

Freedom after seizures doesn't come in a sudden, dramatic moment; it's built through daily choices, asking for help, doing some rehab exercises, saying a prayer, taking medication consistently, and celebrating small wins. You have the strength to overcome your fears, and your light can shine through even the darkest times. Don't fight with big gestures, but with the steady, stubborn courage of showing up for your own life, day after day.

Gratitude as Medicine

Lying in that hospital bed, the room transformed into a modest theater of benevolence. Practical actions such as a nurse adjusting my blanket at 3 a.m., a technician dedicating time to clarify why my IV pump was beeping, and a physical therapist celebrating my initial unsteady steps with a humorous high-five exemplified this. However, it was the collective impact of these minor acts that served as an essential form of therapy.

Those moments that stuck with me: the orderly who brought my parents steaming soup when the hospital cafeteria had closed, the coworker who sat with me and scrolled through old photos until I burst into laughter, and the volunteer who brought a puzzle book and stayed long enough to find the first few answers, making me feel capable again. These moments of human warmth made the sterile hours more bearable.

What stayed with me were the sensory details. A colleague's bouquet, slightly wilted at the edges, filled the room with a faint, sweet fragrance, serving as a quiet, living reminder that people had visited. My phone lit up with text message threads in waves: short, steady bursts "How are you?" "Called HR to sort out the leave," which felt like a sign of support. Friends drove to see me for a few moments, and we sat in the bright waiting room, where everything tasted impossibly good. My family arranged for rotating meals so they wouldn't have to cook for weeks.

Gratitude became a daily habit for me. I kept a small notebook by my bedside named "Tiny Triumphs." On difficult mornings, I'd force myself to write down one thing I was grateful for: maybe a nurse who remembered to adjust my pillow, a voicemail from an old student that made me smile, or the smell of rain coming in through an open window. Those little notes felt like tiny prayers. At night, I'd put my phone face down and spend five minutes saying out loud the names of three people who helped me that day and why. It seemed simple, but this habit changed my outlook; eventually, my eyes started to notice the good things.

There were tough moments that caught me off guard. Some days, the pain lingered longer than anyone expected, and the nausea from medication made eating feel like a chore. I had moments of ugly, private anger - at the unfairness of it all, the lost time, and having to rely on others. On those days, I learned to turn gratitude into honesty, like telling a visiting friend, "I'm sorry I'm short today; I'm grateful you're here even if I'm being a grump." Those honest admissions fostered a more caring kind of support. My sister, who knew my short fuse, would bring quiet company instead of empty words, and a friend who lived nearby would drop everything to run to the pharmacy when I needed a refill, so I didn't have to add that to my to-do list.

What I found helpful was celebrating my small victories out loud, like texting, "Today I made it a short shower!" because acknowledging those achievements helped others share in my happiness and boosted my own confidence that I was moving in the right direction.

Practical ways gratitude helped me heal: Keep a notebook by your bedside to write down one small success each day. Over time, it becomes a testament to your progress. Save messages and cards in a folder to read when you're feeling down. Ask for specific help, like "Can you sit with me for 30 minutes?" or "Can you pick up my groceries?" so others know exactly how to support you. Swap outward thanks for inward permission:

let yourself accept help without feeling guilty, it's part of taking care of each other.

What surprised me most was how gratitude transformed my inner world. Instead of just dealing with pain and fear, I began to notice consistent support I could rely on. Recognizing these supports didn't remove hardship, but it shifted the narrative from "I'm suffering alone" to "I'm being supported." Knowing that people were both literally and figuratively helping carry the burden allowed me to focus on healing. Months later, those initial acts of kindness still create a ripple effect.

As I went through my own experience, I found myself writing thank-you cards and later volunteering to sit with other patients on the same ward. Gratitude became more than just a feeling; it became an action, helping me turn the care I'd received into something that could sustain others. If there's one simple truth I took away from that time, it's this: healing is rarely something you can do on your own. Community, whether it's small acts of kindness or quiet prayers, works like medicine, speeding up recovery in ways that both the body and the heart can understand.

Appreciate every act of kindness, keep a record of small achievements, and let gratitude be the remedy you turn to during tough days. Although it won't eliminate suffering, it will change how you cope with it and the people who support you.

"Courage isn't always loud. Often, it's the soft voice at the end of the day saying, 'I will try again tomorrow.'" — Mary Anne Radmacher

Final Inspiration

To all readers of this book, whether facing health issues, personal setbacks, or uncertain circumstances, I want to share a message that goes beyond simple words of comfort: I speak from the small, everyday moments that quietly lay the groundwork for a renewed life. You have greater resilience than you may realize. Your journey isn't defined only by the challenges you encounter but by how you respond to them. Even in your most vulnerable moments, you carry a steady strength and an unextinguished light.

Resilience is more about daily habits than big gestures. You can see it in the simple act of waking up and taking a full minute to breathe slowly before getting out of bed. It's also found in the quiet moment of sipping a cup of tea and gazing out the window for five minutes, even when you're tempted to rush off.

It's the day you pick up the phone to schedule a follow-up instead of letting fear hold you back. It's taking the stairs when you couldn't do it the day before. Those small, everyday actions, like getting up, brushing your teeth, or walking a block, are the building blocks of recovery. Real life will challenge you in practical, sometimes messy ways. You'll face appointments that drain you, forms that frustrate you, and nights when the pain or sadness feels like clouds closing in. There will be days when twenty minutes of handling work emails feels like a win; celebrate that.

There will be weeks when exhaustion takes over, and you find yourself napping at 3 p.m.; don't be ashamed. You might need to negotiate a reduced schedule, ask a colleague to cover a meeting, or let a friend pick up your groceries. These aren't failures; they're strategies for navigating tough times and emerging stronger. Focus on the people who show up to support you.

Ask directly for what you need: "Can you spare 30 minutes to chat?" "Would you mind running an errand for me?" "Can you remind me to stay hydrated throughout the day?" Most people are willing to help out when they know exactly what to do. Keep a list of who to call for what: a neighbor for groceries, a sibling for rides, a friend for a distraction. Let their presence be a source of strength, not a burden on your pride.

Establish daily rituals that ground you. Keep a small "victory jar" and add a note each time you accomplish something that moves you forward, whether it's a simple task like taking a shower or a short walk. Maintain a bedside notebook where you write down one positive thing that happened each day, no matter how minor. When fear strikes, practice calming techniques by identifying five things you see, four you can touch, three you hear, two you smell, and one you taste. Use a single compassionate phrase to repeat on tough mornings, such as "I'm doing my best today, and that's enough." Break your goals into smaller, achievable steps and keep them visible.

Instead of saying "get better," try setting specific, achievable goals, such as "I'll stand up for five minutes without sitting" or "I'll call the clinic to confirm my appointment." Use a calendar, checklists, or a habit-tracking app to stay on top of your progress. Often, progress is hard to see until you start tracking it, and those small checkmarks add up to show you're moving forward. It's okay to feel sad and angry, but don't let those emotions hold you back. Acknowledge the things you've lost, like your daily routine, energy, independence, or a specific role.

Give yourself space to grieve, then choose one small, restorative action such as calling a friend, reading a chapter, or taking a ten-minute break in the sun. Be gentle with yourself and speak to yourself as you would to someone you care about who's hurting. Remember that change is possible. My recovery wasn't a single, magical moment; it was a series of small wins, like a clear morning, a week without seizures, a lunch with a friend, or a drive down a familiar street.

Everyone has rewritten their story in their own way. Your best days aren't behind you; they can still come if you keep showing up, even if it's just taking one breath at a time or having someone by your side. Ultimately, let your experiences guide your path forward. Share your story when you feel ready; telling it can restore your power and help others too. Offer some of your time when you can, whether it's bringing soup, sitting with someone in the hospital, or sending a message of hope. These small acts create a support circle and boost your healing process.

Don't fear tough times; they help you grow stronger. Believe in yourself. Be grateful for those who support you. Celebrate each small achievement. Your future remains open, ready to be shaped by your strength and story. Keep moving forward. Stay bright and shining. The light inside you is enough for one intentional breath, one small step, one courageous day at a time.

Despite any challenge you face, your strength, hope, and faith shine brightly. This truth shows in the small, everyday choices you make. It's the hand you reach for when you feel dizzy; the text you send a friend asking for help with groceries; the ten slow breaths you take before answering a tough phone call. These quiet acts are a testament to the unbreakable light inside you, and they add up faster than you might realize. When the path feels overwhelming, turn to practices that make your faith and hope feel real.

Start each day with a steady, intentional ritual: spend a minute doing deep breathing exercises, say a quick prayer, or write a line in your journal recognizing something you're thankful for. Keep a small collection of messages, cards, and photos that you can look back on during tough days, serving as tangible reminders of care that are always nearby. Let routines act as anchors: morning stretches, a brief walk around the block, or a quick call to a loved one.

These actions do not eliminate hardship but offer enough steadiness to keep progressing. Accepting setbacks is key to building strength. Some days, you might move two steps forward and one step back, facing a new pain, a restless night, or a disappointing test result, but such moments do not mean defeat.

Acknowledge the setback, experience the emotions, and then take one small step forward: refill a prescription, schedule a follow-up, or take a break with a cup of tea. Celebrate those tiny choices as victories; they're the foundation of lasting recovery and renewal. Faith and hope are also community-based. Let others help in specific ways: ask a neighbor to pick up a prescription, a sibling to sit with you while you tackle a tough task, or a friend to bring a meal. Be clear about what you need so others can lend a hand without having to guess. And when you're able, pay it forward with a short note, a listening ear, or a shared meal because giving back strengthens your own heart.

Don't forget to recognize the small victories: a peaceful night's sleep, a conversation that lingers, a short, steady walk. These moments show that your inner light isn't just shining but growing brighter. Keep trusting in yourself. Be grateful for every small step forward. The future is yours to shape, and your best days are still ahead, ready for you to meet with one brave, everyday step.

"Never give up, for that is just the place and time that the tide will turn." — Harriet Beecher Stowe

Live with courage, trust the process, and keep shining your light; you can conquer anything. Below, I've broken down how the practices you mentioned, meditation, staying calm, trusting your medical team, and expressing gratitude, played out in everyday, real-life ways during my journey, and how others can apply them too.

Meditation and brief mindfulness practices

Start your day with a 3-minute morning ritual: lie in bed, place one hand on your chest, breathe in for 4 counts, hold for 2 counts, and exhale for 6 counts. Do this three times before getting up to calm your nervous system. Throughout the day, take 60-second micro-meditations: sit quietly and focus on a single breath in and out. You can also use a guided 5–10 minute app session (either breath-focused or body-scan) before your appointments. Before procedures, visualize a favorite place in vivid detail - imagine the smell of the ocean, the warmth of the sun on your skin.

Practicing calming scenes before medical procedures like MRI, EEG, or surgery can help reduce anxiety. Try counting your breaths while waiting for tests or repeating a calming mantra in your mind during IV insertions or scans. To stay calm during real-life medical moments, prepare the night before by packing a small bag with cozy clothes, hand lotion, noise-canceling earbuds, a list of questions, ID, insurance information, and a picture of someone you love. Having familiar items with you can help keep you grounded.

Try the "pause-and-plan" technique: when fear rises, take a moment to pause, name your feelings aloud ("I'm feeling scared"), breathe slowly a few times, and pick one quick action (like calling your spouse, asking a nurse a question, or sipping water). Turning emotion into action can help lessen overwhelm. Having someone with you who understands your calming signals (such as squeezing your hand to slow down or using a practiced phrase to signal silence) can be really helpful. Practical distractions like playlists, audiobooks, or reading a familiar prayer, psalm, or scripture out loud while waiting can also help keep you steady during long clinic days.

Building trust with your medical team is essential. Come prepared with a list of questions for each visit: "What's the goal of this test?" "What are the possible outcomes?" "What should I look for at home?" "Who should I contact if X happens?" Asking clear and specific questions helps build confidence. Keep a notebook for appointments with details such as date, who you saw, key recommendations, medication names and doses, and next steps. This simple approach helps prevent confusion and puts you in control. Also, ask your clinician to explain their plan and then repeat it back to them ("So I'll stop taking medication an on day X, and come back for imaging on Y"). This ensures you understand everything and allows them to correct any mistakes.

This helps build shared understanding. When you feel like you're not being heard, try to schedule a brief care conference or ask the most senior clinician to review the plan. Most teams respond well to calm and specific advocacy. Gratitude can be part of a daily routine. Try keeping a "Tiny Triumphs" jar: write down one small achievement each day and place it in the jar (like taking a shower, having a pain-free hour, or receiving a visit). On tough days, take a moment to read some of the slips aloud. You can also try a nightly gratitude check-in: name three specific things that happened that day you are thankful for (like a friendly nurse, a kind message from a neighbor, or a warm cup of tea).

Being specific makes gratitude more concrete. Pay it forward by sending a quick thank-you note or voice message to someone who lent a hand whenever you can. Showing appreciation strengthens your connection and gives you a sense of empowerment. Practical coping habits that helped me move forward include breaking tasks into small, manageable steps. Instead of saying "get better," set specific goals like "stand up for five minutes," "walk to the end of the block," or "make a call to the clinic." Celebrate each milestone as a win. Track your progress with a simple calendar or checklist. Seeing visual evidence of repeated small wins boosts your confidence. For better sleep, limit screen time an hour before bed, dim the lights, and practice slow breathing to help you fall asleep.

Even small improvements in sleep can significantly boost resilience. Nutrition and hydration can be just as vital as medication. Keep a water bottle nearby, ask for your favorite foods if hospital meals aren't appealing, and consider accepting meal trains at home to reduce decision fatigue. When setbacks occur, expect plateaus and temporary challenges, such as extra pain days, imaging delays, or medication side effects. During these times, take a step back, acknowledge the setback, reach out for support, rest, and identify a small next step to try. Keep a list of questions for your healthcare team and bring it to appointments so setbacks become opportunities for troubleshooting rather than spiraling into worries.

Here are some concrete phrases that have helped me and can help you too: "What's the plan if this happens again?" (for contingency planning) "I need a minute to myself; can you give me two minutes?" (setting boundaries) "I'm feeling overwhelmed; can you repeat that and spell out the medication?" (clarity) "Can you remind me why we're doing this test?" (reorientation)

Inspirational Message and Quote

"The only way to find out what's possible is by trying what seems impossible."

Regardless of the challenges you face, whether it's a medical diagnosis, a long recovery, a career setback, or anxiety about the future, remember that resilience is both practical and spiritual. Strength often shows not in grand gestures but through small, consistent actions that build up over time. Here are realistic, everyday strategies that bring the essence of this quote into daily life: start with tiny steps. On tough days, progress might just be making a cup of coffee, brushing your teeth, or walking to the end of the driveway. These small victories help rebuild confidence and momentum.

Keep a visible checklist to monitor your progress. Cultivate a habit of focusing on hope. Begin each morning with a one-minute breathing exercise, a quick prayer, or a few lines of gratitude in a bedside journal. These small rituals help anchor you when the world feels overwhelming. Prepare for the medical and practical parts of your situation. Pack a bag for appointments with essentials like glasses, a list of questions, a picture of someone you care about, and a notebook. Use a single notebook to track medications, follow-ups, and insurance calls, making sure you don't overlook any important details.

Building small organizational habits can help lower stress and enable you to take proactive steps instead of just reacting. Reach out to your support network. Be clear about what you need from others, such as asking a friend to pick up your prescription or sit with you while you make a call. This allows friends and family to offer meaningful support. Asking for help isn't a sign of weakness; it's a strategic part of recovery that relies on teamwork. Turn your emotions into action. When fear becomes too much to handle, recognize it: "That's fear." Then, choose a physical activity to focus on, such as drinking water, standing up and stretching, or making a phone call. By converting your emotions into action, you can break the cycle of helplessness.

Embrace adaptive patience. Expect setbacks, such as bad nights, delays, or side effects, and plan for small adjustments: rest, a quick favorite distraction, or one action to follow up on the next day. View setbacks as bumps in the road, not as insurmountable obstacles. Find your identity through tiny daily rituals. If your work, hobbies, or social roles feel out of reach, reconnect with them in small ways: respond to one email, read a page of a book, or sketch for a few minutes. These small acts can help you reconnect with your true self. Recognize and celebrate your progress. Save messages, cards, and photos from the people who've supported you.

When you're having a tough day, re-reading these words serves as a powerful reminder that you're not alone and that you've overcome challenges before. Find meaning in your struggles. Take a moment each week to write down what you've learned - maybe it's gaining patience, setting clearer priorities, or building stronger relationships. Creating meaning doesn't eliminate the pain, but it can transform your experiences into a source of strength for the future. Life is messy, and that's okay. Appointments will run late, your energy will fluctuate, and your emotions will rise and fall.

Nevertheless, attempting what appears to be impossible, such as resuming a normal activity, confronting a test result, or requesting the assistance necessary, begins with a single, intentional, and routine step.

Your courage is demonstrated not through a single monumental act but through the cumulative effect of numerous small, courageous decisions. Maintain your confidence in yourself. Remain optimistic and pragmatic. Cling to hope, take the subsequent small step, and trust that brighter days are being shaped by the consistent actions you undertake today.

Chapter 5:
Recovery and Rehabilitation

The Physical and Emotional Journey

A Path of Resilience, Trust, and Transformation

Recovering from brain surgery is not merely about physical healing; it's a complex journey that involves patience, resilience, and hope. I aim to share my experience not as a medical professional but as someone who has navigated this path with courage and conviction. I emphasize that recovery can be transformative despite obstacles and setbacks, revealing strengths and insights that we may not have recognized within ourselves.

Trusting the Process: A Personal Reflection

After leaving the hospital following surgery, I felt a mixture of relief and cautious hope. The successful procedure marked an important milestone, showing that I had made significant progress in overcoming the persistent seizures that had once defined my life. Still, I understood that my journey was just beginning. Like life itself, recovery demands patience, resilience, and unwavering trust.

For several weeks after the surgical procedure, I remained under close supervision, constantly monitored by a dedicated team of medical professionals, including doctors, nurses, and specialists. Their expertise and compassionate care reassured me and served as a profound reminder of the importance of trusting the healing process. Each day, I received prescriptions for antibiotics to prevent infection, anti-inflammatory medications to reduce swelling, and pain relievers to ease discomfort. I reclined in bed, fully aware of the pain with each movement and mindful of the fragility of my physical condition. During these moments, I practiced gratitude, giving thanks to God for His blessings, the skilled hands of the medical team, and the opportunity to recover.

The mental and emotional aspects of recovery, arguably the most difficult part, also started to emerge. I struggled with feelings of frustration and helplessness. Tasks that once seemed simple, like getting out of bed, walking short distances, and dressing, became major challenges. The simple act of holding a spoon or standing without support felt as hard as climbing a mountain. In those moments, I understood a basic truth: patience was a virtue and my lifeline.

Emotionally, the beginning of my recovery was profoundly humbling. Tasks that were once simple, such as walking to the bathroom, dressing, or brushing my teeth, now require great effort and sometimes assistance. I had to rethink what progress meant, shifting it from productivity to persistence. Every small act of independence became a milestone.

The frustration I experienced was genuine at times. Sometimes, I felt like crying, and I would occasionally give in to the urge. However, I reminded myself every day: *"This is a journey, not a race."* With that mindset, I continued forward—step by step, breath by breath.

I committed to approaching each day with the mindset: **"This is a journey, not a race."** I continually reminded myself that progress is incremental and setbacks are a natural part of the growth process. Each small victory, standing unaided, taking a few steps, eating without assistance, became a testament to resilience, built piece by piece.

The Strength of Physical Rehabilitation and Inner Resilience

Physical therapy became a daily routine that helped rebuild my confidence and strength. I clearly remember the first time I tried lifting a small weight, an effort that seemed minor but felt like a major breakthrough. My muscles trembled, and every small improvement felt like overcoming a challenge. With each session, I gradually pushed my boundaries by lifting lighter weights, doing slow, controlled repetitions, and steadily restoring my unrestricted movement.

There were times of doubt when I felt overwhelmed and frustrated by the slow recovery or pain that seemed greater than my effort. Still, I kept going. I realized resilience is built not just in moments of strength but also through perseverance during tough times. My journey proved that progress, no matter how slow, still counts as real progress. Both my body and mind were opening to new possibilities.

The Emotional Terrain: Confronting Inner Undercurrents

My emotional state during recovery was as turbulent as the physical healing process. I experienced feelings of vulnerability, mild depression, and occasional despair. I learned that it's normal to feel overwhelmed, especially when simple tasks like walking or dressing seem impossible. However, I found that honestly acknowledging these feelings was freeing. Sharing my thoughts with trusted friends, family, or a professional psychologist gave me an outlet for my emotions. This openness greatly eased my burden.

Practicing mindfulness and maintaining a positive outlook proved vital. Focusing on the present moment rather than dwelling on losses or unachieved goals helped me find deep tranquility. I realized the powerful link between the mind and body: mental resilience has a significant impact on physical healing. Building hope and confidence, even from small achievements, motivated me to keep moving forward.

Milestones of Development: Rekindling Self-Reliance

Coming back to the gym after nearly a year and a half was a deeply rewarding step in my recovery. I started with light weights and slow reps, gradually rebuilding my strength. What initially felt like simple lifting and movement turned into a powerful act of reclaiming my independence. Each small improvement felt like a quiet victory over obstacles.

A Stoic Letter to You, the One Seeking Strength

To You, the One Walking the Path of Strength

Every day, you face a world that isn't always fair or kind. Still, you get up every morning. That **in itself** is an achievement.

Avoid seeking comfort in praise or hiding within routines. The Stoic understands that true **greatness is forged through struggle**, not ease.

If today presents challenges — good, as it's you're training.

If others test your patience — good, as it's your discipline.

If you're tired, good, as it's an opportunity to practice endurance.

Nothing is denied to you except what was never meant for you to control.

"You have power over your mind — not outside events. Realize this, and you will find strength."

So don't wish for events to go your way. Instead, wish to be **worthy of any event.**

Stand as the rock that waves crash against — unmoved, unmoved, unmoved.

Daily Stoic Affirmation for You:

"I cannot control what happens — but I command how I respond. I choose calm. I choose strength. I choose virtue."

Your Daily Stoic Morning Routine

(5–10 minutes)

1. Morning Intention

Say aloud or write:

Today, I will focus on practicing one of the following: courage, patience, discipline, humility, acceptance, or resilience.

Example:

Today, I choose to practice **discipline**, no matter how I feel. It's a small step, but it's a step toward growth and consistency.

2. Stoic Affirmation (Repeat 3x)

"I cannot control what happens — but I command how I respond. I choose calm. I choose strength. I choose virtue."

3. Read or Reflect on a Stoic Quote

Choose one each day. Here are some options you can rotate through:

- **Marcus Aurelius:**

  "The impediment to action advances action. What stands in the way becomes the way."

- **Epictetus:**

  "We suffer more often in imagination than in reality."
- **Seneca:**

  "He who is brave is free."

4. One-Minute Silent Reflection

Remain seated. Take a deep breath. Reflect thoughtfully.

"What events could I face today? How can I respond with virtue?"

This creates **emotional resilience even** before the day starts.

5. Write this prompt in a journal (optional)

What kind of person will I choose to be today, no matter what the world is like?

Even a single sentence can have a profound impact. Simply write truthfully.

Chapter 6:
Life After Brain Surgery: Adapting to New Realities and Finding Myself Again

Rebuilding, Rediscovering, and Embracing a New Beginning

After regaining consciousness in the Intensive Care Unit, a new chapter unfolded, characterized by hope, vulnerability, and resilience. The room had a peaceful, almost meditative quality, disturbed only by the soft hum of monitors and the rhythmic beeping representing life's heartbeat. I vividly remember a strange mix of feelings: a dull pain combined with mild nausea from anesthesia, and a fog that blurred my vision, making the surroundings feel distant yet oddly familiar. My body was heavy, as if cocooned in fragile delicacy.

My parents, family, and friends were crucial to my recovery. My father traveled all the way from the Dominican Republic, crossing oceans and mountains, out of love and duty to support me during this critical period. His consistent presence provided strength, filling the space with warmth and reassurance. He was there during that vulnerable time and remained with me through the entire recovery process—attending therapy sessions, encouraging every small step, and sharing quiet moments of hope and resilience. My mother, too, after work, always took care of me.

I truly appreciate, from the bottom of my heart, all the sacrifices made to care for me throughout my recovery. To my family and friends, thank you for always being there for me. To my readers, I encourage you to cherish your family, even during challenging times like surgery and recovery; they will always be there. A friend or coworker who becomes like family through love and care also counts; it doesn't have to be blood relation. Love yourself first, but also love your loved ones as I love you.

My father's support lifts my spirits and strengthens my resolve to heal. I also see how vital his constant presence was to my mother, who tirelessly supports our family and finds comfort knowing that her two greatest treasures share strength. Their combined support creates an environment of love and steady hope, guiding my path to recovery and reminding me that I was never alone in this challenge.

The simple yet powerful memory of seeing him remains with me forever. It reminds me that, no matter how lonely or fragile we feel during life's toughest moments, family love and steadfast support are our anchors. I experienced deep gratitude and calming reassurance, realizing I was not alone. This was a second chance to persevere, live more fully, unlock my potential, and slowly restore my life.

The First Weeks of Recovery: Patience, Trust, and Small Victories

In the following days, I participated in a delicate dance of recovery, a continuous journey of healing encompassing much more than just physical aspects. I remained in the hospital for several weeks, under the attentive care of a dedicated team of doctors, nurses, and specialists who skillfully guided my recovery. Each morning, I was awakened by the soft footsteps of nurses who checked my vital signs, adjusted my medications, and encouraged me to manage the discomfort through deep breathing.

Medications were essential for my recovery, including antibiotics to prevent infection, anti-inflammatory drugs to reduce swelling, and pain relievers to ease the constant ache throughout my head and body. The discomfort felt like a dull, unyielding drumbeat in my skull, always reminding me of my physical state. However, the biggest daily challenge I faced was patience.

Although medications supported my body, it was the intentional strategies I adopted that supported my mind. I understood early on that I needed more than just rest; I required a rhythm of resilience and a structure of hope to get through the toughest days. Each morning, even when lifting my head was painful, I would whisper or write:

Today, I will focus on practicing: [select one — courage, patience, discipline, humility, acceptance, resilience].

Example: "Today, I will focus on practicing discipline no matter how I feel.

It evolved into a sacred routine that set the tone for my day, aligning my thoughts with purpose instead of fear. When I felt vulnerable, I chose acceptance; when I needed to endure therapy or pain, I selected courage. These words served as lightweight armor, protective yet unobtrusive.

Every morning, I begin with a straightforward Stoic affirmation, softly spoken either aloud or in my mind, repeated three times as a personal vow.

I cannot control what happens — but I decide how I respond.

I choose calmness. I choose strength. I choose virtue.

The more I repeated it, the more it embedded itself in my thoughts. It became a quiet act of defiance against despair, a statement that, although my body might have felt broken, my spirit stayed whole. I may have lost control of many things, but my character remained intact. This realization alone reignited my sense of dignity, even during vulnerable moments.

Even with painkillers and medication, the most challenging aspect of recovery was developing patience. On some mornings, lifting my arm felt as difficult as moving a massive boulder. Sitting up in bed caused trembling, and standing with help was physically draining. I would concentrate on my feet, hoping they would recall how to move, but often they didn't.

Frustration would sneak in like an uninvited guest, whispering doubts: You're not healing quickly enough. You're failing. However, I countered those thoughts with deliberate reflection, constantly reminding myself:

This is a journey, not a race.

You're not falling behind; you're in the process of becoming.

Some mornings, even simple movements like lifting my arm, sitting up, or standing with help felt overwhelming, like climbing a small mountain. Still, I kept telling myself, **"This is a journey, not a race,"** reminding myself to stay patient. Every small achievement, whether it was taking a few assisted steps, squeezing a hand, or opening my eyes without pain, reflected my resilience and progress.

I realized that true strength builds over time. I steadily progressed, rebuilt trust in my body, and exercised patience during the healing process. This journey was both humbling and empowering. I understood that resilience isn't about rushing recovery, but about recognizing my limits and valuing the path of personal growth, learning each lesson along the way. It's not just about healing, but also about personal and professional development, which is a powerful tool to acquire.

The Inner Journey: A Path to Emotional Healing and Self-Balance

Recovery transcended mere physical strength; it represented a profound exploration into the deeper aspects of my being, challenging perceptions of vulnerability and frustration that at times threatened to overwhelm me. There were moments when I encountered despair, as the frustration of being unable to perform tasks with the ease and confidence I once had loomed over me. I would sit in my hospital bed, gazing at the ceiling, the discomfort in my muscles reflecting a deep yearning for independence, normalcy, and meaning.

Every small act, like squeezing a hand, blinking without pain, or sitting a bit longer than the previous day, felt like a victory. I began a Progress Journal not to record perfection but to honor perseverance. One entry stated:

I managed to stand on my own for eight seconds today. Afterwards, I cried not from pain, but because of a personal accomplishment.

These small steps were no mere actions; they laid the groundwork for something greater: trust. I started to regain trust in my body, and even more crucially, I started to trust myself again.

Therapy sessions had a strict structure, but what benefited me most was setting a clear mental intention before each one. I would take deep breaths and remind myself:

I'm here to grow and try. I'm not limited by what I can't do today; I'm defined by my commitment to keep showing up. Some days, I practiced courage. Others, I needed humility. And often, I practiced acceptance, not giving up, but choosing peace over resistance.

The inner journey, his silent quest for emotional healing, proved to be even more difficult than the physical one. I experienced times of deep vulnerability, where tears flowed not only from pain but from feeling trapped in a body that once moved easily. There were many long nights when the gentle hum of fluorescent lights reflected the solitude of recovery.

Even during the quietest times, I discovered strength. I vowed not to let these moments shape me but to use them to improve. I followed a straightforward rule:

When you're feeling uncertain, concentrate on acts that benefit your future self.

I envisioned a future version of myself walking again, laughing without fear, running, dancing, and living free from constant discomfort. This vision guided me. I started writing letters, notes, and journaling to that future self, keeping them in a notebook. Each letter was labeled with a date, such as "Read this on your first walk outside" or "For the day you no longer need painkillers." These notes became promises, my personal vows of perseverance.

One of the notes mentioned:

Dear future me:

If you're reading this, you've broken through the fog. Remember the strength it took to rise when no one was watching. That same strength still lives inside you. Never forget what it took to become whole again, and perhaps the most important lesson? I realized **resilience isn't flashy.** It doesn't always make a lot of noise. Sometimes, resilience is a quiet choice to try *again*, push a little further, breathe through another wave of pain, or smile even when your body doesn't feel like it.

The hospital room became a sanctuary, a space for renewal rather than confinement, and honestly, it became a second home to me. Each day, my wounds shifted from feeling like a burden to becoming part of my growth. I was being shaped not into my old self but into a person who is more profound, more conscious, and more alive. Now, I carry these strategies with me, simple yet powerful practices that keep me grounded.

Begin your day by setting an intention:
"Today I will focus on courage, discipline, patience..."

- **Repeat your Stoic affirmation:** "I cannot control what happens — but I command how I respond."

- **Celebrate small victories: Maintain a journal and record every bit of progress. Every detail counts.**

- **Visualize your future self:** embody the person you are becoming.

- **Write notes to yourself:** Remind yourself of who you are on days you forget.

I realized that recognizing these emotions was not a sign of weakness but a vital part of healing. I reached out for support by sharing my feelings with loved ones and having open conversations with a psychologist, who helped me explore the complexities of my experiences. Mindfulness became an important tool; I practiced deep breathing and focused on the present, avoiding dwelling on the past or the uncertain future. Over time, I shifted my mindset, replacing feelings of helplessness with gratitude for my small wins and the progress I made.

Chapter 7:
Inspiration and Hope: Gaining Resilience Through Challenges

Living with epilepsy is like riding tumultuous waves, marked by episodes of despair and surprising bursts of strength. Looking back on my journey, I see how these painful yet triumphant moments have shaped who I am today. This story transcends medical treatments; it celebrates the resilience of the human spirit, the determination to overcome obstacles, and the hope that sustains us during challenging times.

The Difficulties of an Unpredictable Journey Looking back on those early years, I remember sleepless nights filled with anxiety about the looming seizures, uncertain if I would wake up shrouded in confusion or exhaustion. My body shook, my throat tightened with fear, and my mind swirled with unspoken questions.

The seizures hit like sudden storms, overwhelming with their abruptness and leaving me exhausted, physically and emotionally. I see how these painful, yet triumphant moments have shaped who I am. This story isn't just about medicine and surgery; it's a tribute to the human spirit. It highlights the invisible strength we all possess, the quiet voice encouraging us to "try again" when we feel like giving up. This is a tale of resilience and perseverance in the face of difficulties, and the enduring light of hope even in our darkest nights.

There were many times I felt sidelined, observing life as fragments that seemed detached and incomplete. The substantial risks I faced caused me to miss out on family vacations and special moments that should have brought joy and relaxation. I yearned to be with friends, participating in activities like cycling, going to the beach, and discovering new places. Yet, my condition constantly overshadowed these simple joys. At times, I felt ashamed of my inability to fully engage; other times, I felt powerless, caught in a cycle beyond my control.

Discovering the Flame Within

Even during the darkest and most turbulent times, a small, persistent part of me refused to fade away a tiny, unwavering flicker of hope that persisted, even when nearly overwhelmed by despair.

I view every setback not as a form of punishment, but as an opportunity for preparation.

Every seizure, hospital visit, and limitation contributed to my growth, shaping who I am. I began to question: What is this experience teaching me? Who am I becoming because of it? Amidst the pain, I discovered my inner strength, gentle, unassuming, yet resilient.

As the Stoics say, "The obstacle in your path becomes the path forward." The very challenges that threatened to defeat me ultimately strengthened me. It was no longer about the seizures. Instead, it was about how I decided to use what I had been given.

Amidst this turmoil, something remarkable appeared: a steadfast glimmer of hope that refused to fade. I remained convinced that even during the bleakest times, when seizures continued endlessly and the future felt uncertain, I possessed a core of resilience. I saw challenges as opportunities, lessons concealed in hardship, but vital for growth.

Viewing Challenges as Opportunities for Growth

My defining moment occurred when I chose to undergo surgery, a courageous step that changed my life. I remember the days leading up to the operation: the many consultations and sleepless nights spent thinking about my future. In 2008, I had a different surgery for my right shoulder injuries, which included a fracture and dislocation of both shoulders. I also have two screws in my right shoulder from a seizure triggered while I watched a 3D movie at the theater. For some people with epilepsy, watching 3D movies or shows can trigger seizures, not all of course, but for some, it can trigger an episode, so keep that in mind, fellow epilepsy community. This experience showed my ability to face physical trauma and emerge stronger. It taught me that healing often requires patience, humility, and courage.

This time, the stakes were much higher. The surgery involved complex neurological work, specifically removing scar tissue from my hippocampus to prevent disruptive electrical activity. My medical team explained the risks, expected results, and the importance of staying hopeful. I looked at MRI scans showing dark, textured scars in my brain that had caused years of turmoil. Sitting in that hospital room, I consciously chose to trust the process, embracing faith and resilience, knowing the outcome could be life-changing.

The Journey Towards Physical and Emotional Recovery

In the days immediately after my surgery, I experienced a fragile balance. The hospital served as a space for recovery, with each breath and movement embodying my resolve. The healthcare team, nurses, doctors, and specialists acted as my anchors, thoroughly explaining each step, milestone, and setback. I understood that healing is a nonlinear journey; progress often happens in small, sometimes hardly noticeable, steps.

Physical therapy became my daily lifeline. I would lie back on the bed, my muscles stiff from weeks of immobility, gradually working to restore my strength and mobility. The first time I lifted a lightweight, I felt a surge of pride that reflected my resilience. Gradually, I increased the number of repetitions, pushed through discomfort, and celebrated each small victory, gaining the ability to stand unassisted, take a few cautious steps, and ultimately return to the gym.

Emotionally, I faced moments of uncertainty, feeling overwhelmed by newly discovered limitations, experiencing frustration from setbacks, and expressing concern about the future. Nonetheless, each challenge taught me valuable lessons about the importance of patience. I began to understand that true strength is cultivated not through sudden events, but through sustained and consistent effort.

Practices That Sustained Me

I realized that physical strength wasn't enough; I also needed mental resilience. Therefore, I began incorporating small daily habits to build my inner resilience.

Morning Intention Setting:

Every morning, I would either write or verbally say:

"Today, I will focus on practicing courage, patience, discipline, humility, acceptance, or resilience."

Example: "Today, I commit to practicing discipline, regardless of how I feel."

Stoic Affirmation (Repeat 3 times):

I can't control what happens, but I decide how I respond.

I choose calm. I choose strength. I choose virtue."

Visualization of Victory:

I envisioned myself walking freely, laughing with friends, and raising my arms with ease. This mental image motivated my recovery.

Progress Journal:

I recorded every milestone, big or small, from sitting up without help to walking 10 steps.

Letters to My Future Self:

I sent messages such as:

You did it. Continue to rise. This isn't the conclusion of your journey; it's your rebirth.

These practices grounded me. They reminded me every day that my reaction to life was stronger than anything life could throw at me.

Harnessing Inner Power

Over the weeks, my recovery grew deeper, touching not only my body but also my emotions and spirit. I regained my ability to walk more easily, laughed without hesitation, and reconnected with the world no longer as an epilepsy sufferer, but as a testament to resilience.

I came to a surprisingly simple realization:

The fears we face often serve as gateways to discovering our greatest strengths.

Life will always bring challenges: pain, loss, and uncertainty are unavoidable. However, we are not powerless; we have the ability to respond with strength, clarity, and virtue.

Our mind is within our control, and that is the greatest form of freedom we possess.

Final Thoughts: An Invitation to Never Quit

If you're reading this and confronting a mountain—whether it's illness, grief, fear, or failure—remember this:

You are not broken; you are in the process of becoming.

Your challenges do not determine who you are. Instead, it is your bravery that defines you.

Your pain is not the end; it marks the start of your new journey.

You don't need to be completely fearless; simply show up repeatedly. That's the essence of resilience.

As the Stoics advised, we can't always influence what life presents. However, we do have the ability to choose how we respond. It is in this choice that our freedom resides. Our strength is rooted in this mindset.

So, I leave you with this:

Never lose hope or stop trying.

Your story continues. Your strength remains. Your light continues to shine.

And when you feel at your weakest, remember:

That's when you are being shaped into an unstoppable person.

Chapter 8:
Conquering Insecurity and Accepting Myself

For years, I carried a silent, often hidden burden, an insecurity that quietly affected every part of my life. Living with epilepsy exposed me to a constant sense of vulnerability, leading to doubts about myself and lowering my self-esteem. This shadow grew darker during my teenage years and early adulthood, making me feel inadequate, worthless, and desperate for acceptance as my authentic self. It wasn't only the seizures that troubled me; my self-image played a major role in my inner battles.

I recall gazing at my reflection in the bedroom mirror during those challenging days, as if it were yesterday. My eyes searched for reassurance that I was enough, but all I saw was a young man marked in ways I couldn't understand at the time, someone who felt broken or flawed because of my condition. A part of my identity seemed fragile, as if it could break at any moment, leaving me vulnerable in ways I couldn't always handle.

I remember times when I felt lonely and overwhelmed by self-doubt. My heart would race, and my thoughts would spin into negativity: *Am I lovable? Can anyone truly accept this part of me?* I faced rejection from others and internal doubts, convincing myself that my kindness, care, and integrity were not enough or even signs of weakness. Often, I encountered misunderstandings or rejection when I tried to share my struggles, feelings, or seek support. Some interpreted my compassion as helplessness; others withdrew, lacking empathy and fearing the unknown. These moments of rejection, whether brief or prolonged, deeply affected my self-esteem.

The primary feeling was a sense of being misunderstood and isolated. I felt invisible, even amidst the world's chaos. My confidence waned as I doubted whether I would ever find someone who could love me despite my imperfections and struggles. The desire for real connection turned into a longing that often seemed unreachable, like a distant star I could see but not reach. I questioned if I would ever be enough to be loved, to belong, and to be truly understood.

During difficult times, I often wondered, "Why me?" I reached out with sincere desperation to the universe and God. I tried to shake off doubts that lingered like an unwelcome shadow. Despite showing kindness, respect, and honesty, I felt these qualities were not enough in a society that judges by surface appearances. The internal battle persisted as I questioned my worth, my right to happiness, and whether my scars—both visible and invisible—would always be barriers.

Yet, a gentle and consistent whisper of truth emerged from the darkness, showing that every struggle, rejection, and pain was not a punishment but an essential lesson on my journey to self-acceptance.

The Turning Point: Recognizing My Inner Strength

During instances of despair, I came to the realization that **my insecurity was merely an illusion fashioned by my fears and perceptions, rather than an accurate depiction of my actual reality.** I understood that I possess the inner strength necessary to amend my personal narrative. I have learned that true strength does not lie in dismissing vulnerabilities, but in confronting them with courage and electing to grow despite their presence.

One day, I decided to start a simple journey of self-reconnection. I read books about self-love and resilience, realizing that I was not alone in my experiences; in fact, millions of people around me and worldwide face similar feelings of inadequacy. It was comforting to recognize that self-doubt is a universal challenge, something everyone goes through at some point, regardless of their level of success or confidence.

I began practicing mindfulness meditation, dedicating ten minutes every morning to sit quietly, breathe deeply, and observe my thoughts without any judgment. I became aware of the critical voice that subtly suggested, "You're not enough," and intentionally replaced it with affirmations like, "I am worthy," "I am enough," and "I deserve love." Gradually, these affirmations became part of my inner dialogue, creating a new default mindset.

Gratitude proved to be a powerful practice. Every morning, I paused to appreciate what I had: my health, my family's love, and the small wins

I achieved that day. Sometimes, it was just about the simple act of getting out of bed.

I would like to share some tried-and-true strategies, exercises, and actions that I recommend and have personally practiced.

Techniques and Activities for Building Self-Love and Confidence

Daily affirmations:

Every morning, stand in front of the mirror and say positive affirmations such as:

I deserve love and respect.

My circumstances do not define my worth.

"I am kind, compassionate, and deserving of joy."

Establish this as a daily habit: communicate with confidence and convey authenticity in your interactions.

Journaling Achievements:

Document three achievements each day. Recognize small victories, such as expressing your opinion, smiling, or releasing negative thoughts. Ultimately, these minor successes substantially enhance your self-confidence.

Limit negative self-talk.

Be mindful of instances when self-criticism arises. Substitute "I can't" with "I will try" or "I am enough." Extend the same kindness to yourself that you would offer to a close friend.

Cultivate a mindset focused on growth:

Engage with books or podcasts on personal development. Treat new knowledge and challenges as opportunities to grow. Keep in mind that setbacks are part of the journey, not the end.

Surround yourself with encouraging and positive people.

Engage with friends and family who inspire and uplift your spirit. Avoid negativity and those who undermine your self-esteem.

Develop a self-care routine:

Set aside time for activities that bring you joy, such as exercising, meditating, reading, or engaging in your hobbies. Prioritizing self-care enhances your self-esteem.

Visualize Your Practice:

Picture yourself radiating confidence and happiness while embracing your uniqueness. Let yourself experience these feelings as they come up in the moment. Engage in this practice every day to reinforce your positive beliefs.

Define Personal Objectives:

Divide your dreams into small, manageable actions. Completing each one boosts your confidence and moves you nearer to the life you imagine.

My Journey of Self-Discovery:

Reflecting on my experiences, I've observed a close link between my insecurities and how I see myself. In dating, my kindness sometimes appears to be a weakness. I've encountered many rejections, some taking advantage of my compassion and failing to recognize my true worth. This has led me to reassess my self-esteem and explore the origins of my persistent emotional struggles.

Every setback and heartbreak has served as a valuable lesson. These experiences have shown me that my kindness, respect, and compassion are strengths, not weaknesses. I understand that I don't need validation from others to know my worth; self-confidence is crucial. Supported by my faith, reading, and proactive decisions, I started to see myself in a more positive light. I have learned to embrace my scars, my journey, and my uniqueness. This surgical experience prompted a deeper reflection on my life and led to a significant shift in my mindset.

I now have increased confidence and greet each day with optimism. I approach opportunities with certainty, often thinking, "Yes, I can." Insecurity no longer blocks my path; instead, I channel it into motivation to develop strength, wisdom, and resilience.

Remember: To achieve change, begin now and maintain your focus on discipline.

Life offers numerous challenges alongside moments of beauty and abundance. Your path to overcoming insecurity starts with one step today. Adopt these strategies, believe in your worth, and dedicate yourself to self-love. As you grow more confident, you unlock your potential and shine in ways you've never imagined.

You can make meaningful changes in your life. Your scars, challenges, and experiences are vital parts of your story and contribute to your unique beauty. Accept these aspects, cultivate profound self-love, and consistently work towards your goals. The best version of yourself is on the verge of emerging.

Final Encouragement Note:

It's important to realize that a person's worth isn't determined by others' opinions or past struggles. Each person possesses inherent value, unique qualities, and the ability to achieve any goal they pursue. Every difficulty, rejection, and self-doubt presents an opportunity for growth, strength, and resilience.

Believe in your ability to change, fully embrace self-love, and accept your true self. This confidence will help you overcome any obstacles. No matter the challenges, stay firm in your belief in yourself, as you have an innate strength to conquer even major difficulties.

Today begins your journey to self-love and confidence. Celebrate your unique qualities, take control of your story, and trust that better days are on the horizon. You possess the potential for great accomplishments, and the world awaits to see the extraordinary person you are meant to become.

Final Quote and Confirmation:

Quote:

You possess more bravery than you believe, more strength than you appear to show, and more intellect than you give yourself credit for."

— A.A. Milne.

Confirmation:

Today, I am committed to recognizing my inherent worth. I deserve love, respect, and happiness. I can grow and remain true to my authentic self without wavering. I am unique, empowered, and capable in my own right. I believe in my journey and am confident that better days are ahead. I am prepared to excel and lead a fulfilling life, as I am firmly dedicated to my aspirations.

Chapter 9:
Everyday Struggles We All Encounter

Living with epilepsy frequently entails numerous physical and emotional challenges. It is common to experience feelings of being overwhelmed, frustration, or hopelessness at times, as one navigates emotional fluctuations that may undermine confidence and lead to self-doubt. However, I wish to present a different viewpoint: despite these adversities, each individual possesses distinct strengths. Our conditions should not define our capabilities or impose limitations on us.

Our mental health and emotional well-being are the cornerstones of a happy, fulfilling life. They shape how we see ourselves, connect with others, and navigate the world. When we're emotionally balanced and mentally healthy, we tend to make choices that match our values and goals, and we're more resilient in the face of life's ups and downs. But finding this balance can be tough, especially with the many biological, psychological, and environmental factors that affect our mental state.

A fundamental consideration is the profound interconnection between mental health and physical health. Disruptions in hormonal balance resulting from menopause, thyroid dysfunction, stress, or lifestyle factors can markedly influence mood, energy levels, and overall emotional stability. For example, hormonal fluctuations frequently lead to symptoms such as irritability, anxiety, or sadness, which may be erroneously interpreted as personal shortcomings or a lack of resilience. However, these symptoms are predominantly rooted in biological changes that lie beyond conscious control.

Neurological conditions such as epilepsy, traumatic brain injuries, or neurochemical imbalances can also disrupt normal brain activity, leading to a range of emotional and behavioral symptoms. For example, people with epilepsy may experience mood swings, fear, or confusion during seizures. Some might develop depression or anxiety due to their condition or the medication they're taking to manage it. These experiences can be isolating and overwhelming, but it's important to remember that they are a result of a medical condition, not a personal failing or a lack of strength. Conditions like insomnia, chronic fatigue, or sensory sensitivities can also worsen emotional struggles, making daily life more difficult.

It's a strong reminder that mental health issues often have real physical causes and addressing them requires a caring and comprehensive approach. Seeking help from healthcare professionals, whether through medication, therapy, or lifestyle changes, is an essential step toward reaching stability and recognizing that these struggles are valid and acknowledged. The full spectrum of emotions we experience, from happiness to sadness, is a natural part of being human. It's normal to feel down after a loss, anxious in uncertain situations, or angry when facing injustice. These feelings serve important purposes they alert us to problems that need attention or action.

Still, it's crucial not to let these emotions define who we are or overshadow our sense of self. For many people, feeling deeply is both a blessing and a struggle, particularly when emotions become too much or stick around, leading to conditions like depression or severe anxiety disorders. Recognizing these feelings is a key part of the healing process. Ignoring or pushing them down often exacerbates the pain, while accepting and understanding them can pave the way for growth and self-compassion.

Creating a safe space is essential, whether that involves practicing mindfulness internally or seeking support from supportive loved ones and mental health professionals externally. This environment allows us to express our feelings without shame or judgment. Being emotionally honest empowers us to take proactive steps toward recovery and resilience. Although tough feelings are part of being human, they don't define our full potential. Even amid emotional turmoil, we have an innate ability to grow, change, and renew.

Our strength resides in our capacity to adapt, learn, and seek support when necessary. No individual is exempt from challenges; however, we all possess the ability to navigate through them with perseverance and hope. Selecting paths that promote our mental and emotional growth is an essential component of this journey. Such choices encompass fostering meaningful relationships, engaging in fulfilling work, pursuing hobbies that energize us, and cultivating environments that inspire and motivate us.

People flourish when they feel connected, have a sense of purpose, and achieve things that matter. When we neglect these aspects, we can end up feeling empty or stuck. In our careers, finding work that aligns with our passions and values can be a significant motivator and source of satisfaction. When our daily tasks feel meaningful, it becomes easier to cope with setbacks and stress. On the other hand, staying in environments that breed negativity or burnout can make mental health issues worse. Taking care of ourselves, whether that's taking breaks, setting boundaries, or seeking professional help, is crucial for building emotional resilience.

Relationships are also crucial. Having supportive friends and family around gives us a sense of belonging and security, which can really help our mental health, even when things get tough. Building and keeping these connections takes effort and being open, but the payoff is emotional stability. On the other hand, being in toxic relationships or feeling isolated can make feelings of despair or anxiety worse. That's why it's essential to nurture healthy relationships and reach out for help when needed. Our surroundings and lifestyle choices also have a big impact on our mental health.

Staying physically active, eating a healthy diet, getting enough sleep, and practicing mindfulness, such as meditation or journaling, can help improve our emotional balance. These habits help regulate hormonal fluctuations, reduce stress, and foster a positive mindset. Keep in mind that mental wellness often takes steady work, not instant solutions. It's also crucial to learn how to bounce back from setbacks.

Perseverance is one of our most valuable assets, an enduring trait that often determines how well we navigate life's ups and downs. As time passes, I've come to realize that resilience isn't just about enduring hardships; it's about bouncing back stronger after setbacks. Every obstacle we face isn't an endpoint, but a chance to grow stronger and wiser. When things get tough, I remind myself that these challenging periods are temporary.

They're a natural part of life, like storms that eventually pass, making way for brighter days. This mindset is key because it helps me focus on what I can learn and adapt, rather than what's lost or overwhelming. I've come to realize I have the inner strength to persevere, even when things seem tough or discouraging. Building a mindset that sees challenges as opportunities for growth, whether mental, spiritual, or emotional, takes deliberate effort and practical strategies. Here are some techniques and exercises that can help build resilience and manage emotions more effectively.

Strategies and Activities for Building Resilience

1. Mindfulness and Grounding Techniques:

Make it a daily habit to practice mindfulness, which helps you better understand your emotions without judging them. Try setting aside five minutes to sit quietly, breathe deeply, and pay attention to your thoughts and feelings. When you're feeling anxious or negative, acknowledge those feelings, then shift your focus to your breath or physical sensations. This technique helps you regulate your emotions and find inner calm.

2. Writing for Self-Reflection:

Keep a journal to track your feelings, triggers, and successes. Review situations that cause anxiety or stress, as well as how you responded. Record your goals and note the environments or activities that help you find balance. Over time, this habit will help you better identify what to avoid and what to pursue in life.

3. Create a positive routine:

Organizing your daily schedule around activities that promote well-being, such as exercise, meditation, reading, or hobbies, is crucial. Establishing a routine helps even out mood swings and gives you a sense of control. For instance, starting your day with positive affirmations, taking a short walk, or spending time in prayer can be really beneficial. Additionally, ending your day with a reflection on what went well is highly recommended.

4. Recognize your surroundings and your relationships with others:

Surround yourself with people who lift your spirits, especially those who offer support and encouragement. Try to minimize negativity and toxic situations in your life. Learn to set boundaries and say no to things that don't bring you joy. Identify the environments, activities, and relationships that make you happy and at peace, and prioritize them.

5. Establish Attainable, Incremental Goals:

Decompose extensive objectives into smaller, more manageable tasks. As you undertake these tasks, you will cultivate confidence and resilience. For example, if your aim is to enhance your health, start with daily walks or establish a nutritious eating plan. It is essential to recognize every accomplishment, regardless of its size.

6. Practice Self-Compassion:

Be kind to yourself when things don't go as planned. Recognize that emotional ups and downs are a natural part of growth and change. If you're feeling overwhelmed, acknowledge that it's okay, you're doing the best you can. Treat yourself with the same understanding and compassion you'd show a close friend.

7. Recognize Your Strengths:

Create a List of Your Strengths and Past Achievements. When you're feeling uncertain or going through difficult times, having a personal list of your strengths and accomplishments can be incredibly beneficial. This list reminds you of your resilience, skills, and the obstacles you've already overcome. It can provide a much-needed confidence boost and fresh perspective, showing you that you've faced hardships before and emerged stronger each time.

Why is this list important?

When you're feeling down, overwhelmed, or uncertain, it's easy to get caught up in negative thoughts or self-criticism. But focusing on your strengths and accomplishments can change your mindset from what's not working to what you've already achieved and the qualities that help you bounce back. Acknowledging your own growth, skills, and determination can help you regain your footing, motivation, and a sense of hope.

How to create this list:

1. Identify Your Strengths Think about the personal qualities that stand out to you, such as being resilient, compassionate, patient, creative, adaptable, disciplined, or empathetic. Remember moments when these qualities truly showed. Consider the skills and talents you've gained, like strong communication, problem-solving, leadership, active listening, or technical abilities. What values and passions motivate you? These could include integrity, kindness, curiosity, or perseverance. These strengths are often overlooked, but they are just as important. To begin, try answering some example prompts: When have I shown resilience in my life? What qualities do friends or colleagues often praise me for? Which skills have I developed through work, school, or life experiences?

2. Showcase Your Past Achievements: Personal Milestones - Key moments of personal growth, overcoming challenges, or developing new habits. Professional Accomplishments - Career advancements, successful projects, recognition, awards, or positive feedback. Overcoming Obstacles: Times you faced hardships, financial struggles, loss, or personal setbacks and persevered. Creative Pursuits - Hobbies, art, writing, sports, or any passion where you showed dedication. Learning and Development - New skills acquired, certifications earned, or areas where you've made significant progress. To get started, consider the following prompts: What are three accomplishments I'm most proud of? When did I turn a tough situation into a learning opportunity? What's some positive feedback or praise I've received in the past?

3. Reflect on Your Resilience. Think about times when you faced setbacks but were able to bounce back. This might include overcoming a breakup, recovering from an illness, finding a new job after losing one, or resolving family conflicts. Identify the qualities that helped you get through those tough times, like determination, resourcefulness, patience, and optimism. Remember that each of these experiences has made you stronger and added to your resilience.

4. Make Your List a Daily Reminder. Keep it somewhere visible, like on your mirror, in a journal, or as a note on your phone. Review it often, especially when you're feeling down or unsure. When things get tough, take a moment to recite the facts from your list aloud. Remind yourself: "I'm strong and resilient. I've faced tough times before and come out stronger."

1. Expand and update regularly. Life is dynamic, and your strengths and achievements develop over time. Consistently incorporate new accomplishments or traits you identify in yourself. Reflect on recent challenges and document how you managed them to bolster your evolving resilience.

More Tips: Write your list in a positive and empowering way. Emphasize what you've achieved, rather than what you're missing. Be specific and detailed in your descriptions. For instance, instead of saying "I'm resilient," try "I bounced back from [specific situation], picked up new skills, and moved forward." Also, include evidence: think of compliments, awards, or results that showcase your strengths.

Remember that your strengths and accomplishments show your resilience, adaptability, and ability to grow. When you feel overwhelmed or discouraged, take a moment to review this list. Let it remind you that you've faced tough times before and emerged stronger and wiser. Your resilience is more than just a trait; it's your most valuable asset, something you can rely on when life gets tough. Trust in it, nurture it, and let it guide you through challenging times.

My illustration:

My surgery has led to significant mental and spiritual growth. It has motivated me to develop greater confidence and perseverance. I am fully dedicated to completing any endeavor, whether it's a project, a goal, or a positive choice for myself. I have also enhanced my ability to recognize environments that support me and those that cause stress or negative thoughts.

For example, I used to think that taking part in thrilling and adventurous activities was good for me; although they were sometimes fun, they didn't last. Now, I prefer peaceful surroundings and calming activities. I've also learned to be kinder to myself when things get tough. Instead, I take a step back, give myself a moment to catch my breath, and remind myself that I'm more than my struggles.

Your Ability to Shine:

While epilepsy and mental health challenges are significant aspects of your story, they do not determine your future. You possess the ability to attain success beyond your current expectations. The obstacles you face can contribute to personal growth, and your resilience constitutes your greatest strength.

Remember:

Don't let your emotions control your actions. You have the power to choose your thoughts, behaviors, and the people and things around you. Every challenge can be a chance to bounce back stronger. You have the inner strength to overcome obstacles and succeed. While life can be tough, it also brings beauty, abundance, and potential. Embrace your journey, grow your mind and spirit, and always hold on to hope. The struggle may be hard, but your strength is just as strong.

Strengthening Perseverance: Always Move Forward

It's crucial to remember that, despite life's challenges, strength and perseverance are key to navigating adversity successfully. This idea is worth repeating because of its importance. Reaching success in any area of life depends not just on talent or luck, but also on resilience and a determination to push through tough times. Every challenge offers a chance to build strength, wisdom, and resolve.

Keep pushing forward, stay focused, and never lose hope. Your breakthrough could be just around the corner, as long as you believe in your ability to take the next step. Trust in your own strength; the moment you decide to persist is when your life truly begins to transform.

Motivational Quote:

The pace of progress is not very important as long as there is a steady commitment to improvement.

Final Notice:

People often show abilities that go beyond what they think of themselves. Challenges are just the start of major breakthroughs. Sticking to your beliefs, pushing through, and not giving up are crucial; your achievements, happiness, and inner peace make every effort worth it. Your path is one of a kind, and your strength will help you reach goals that once seemed impossible.

Don't forget that, despite life's challenges, your strength and perseverance are key to overcoming tough times. I stress this important point often. Success in any field doesn't just depend on talent or luck; it's mainly about resilience and a strong commitment to push through, even when faced with huge obstacles. Every challenge offers a chance for personal growth, gaining wisdom, and building determination.

Chapter 10:
Lessons Learned from Experience

Embracing Life's Journey: An Inspirational Guide to Personal Growth

Life is a complex mix of challenges, experiences, and moments of triumph. For people with conditions like epilepsy, this journey can be overwhelming, marked by uncertainty, fears, and the constant struggle to manage unpredictable symptoms. It's normal to feel frustrated or helpless, especially when dealing with the daily realities of a neurological condition. Yet, among these difficulties lies a chance for deep growth—an opportunity to learn more about yourself and discover new strengths and abilities.

Dealing with epilepsy or any long-term condition teaches lessons that go far beyond just overcoming physical challenges. It fosters resilience, patience, and a deeper understanding of your own mind and body. It can be a powerful catalyst for personal growth, prompting you to explore new paths for self-discovery and redefining what success and happiness mean to you. Many people find that, through their struggles, they develop empathy, compassion, and a greater appreciation for life's small but significant moments.

Going through this experience can also give you a unique sense of inner strength, reminding you that you're more capable than you might have thought. It shows that setbacks aren't the end, but rather a part of the growth process. With a commitment to your well-being, determination to persevere, and a positive attitude, you can transform adversity into an opportunity for growth and change. The stories of people who've faced serious health challenges and gone on to achieve their dreams are a testament to this. Their journeys show that where others see obstacles, you can see possibilities.

This guide aims to help you manage the practical side of living with epilepsy, but also to inspire a deeper transformation of your inner self. It encourages you to think about your strengths, recognize your incredible potential, and open up new paths to fulfillment and purpose. Understanding the Inner Transformation: Living with a condition like epilepsy often raises questions about identity, purpose, and limitations. Yet, these questions can be a starting point for profound self-awareness.

By viewing your journey as a valuable chapter of personal growth, you can learn to navigate your experiences with greater confidence and resilience. This process involves more than just medical management; it requires cultivating an inner mindset rooted in hope, courage, and self-compassion. Practical Steps Toward Growth and Self-Discovery: Embrace Your Unique Journey: Accept your diagnosis as part of your life story, an element that, while challenging, also contributes to your strength and wisdom. Celebrate your resilience in the face of daily uncertainties. Set Personal Goals: Even small, achievable goals such as improving self-care routines, learning new skills, or engaging in hobbies can foster a sense of accomplishment and control.

Connect with supportive communities: Share your experiences with others who get what you're going through. Groups, online forums, and similar networks can offer comfort, inspiration, and practical advice. Take care of yourself: Prioritize your physical and emotional well-being by getting enough rest, eating a balanced diet, practicing relaxation techniques like mindfulness or deep breathing, and seeking professional help when you need it. Foster a positive mindset: Focus on being grateful and using affirmations. Look at what you can do, not what you can't. Celebrate your progress, no matter how small.

Discover Your Passions: Take this opportunity to explore interests or activities that bring you happiness and a sense of purpose. Often, these can spark your passion and lead to new possibilities. Stay Informed and Adaptive: Keep up with the latest developments in your condition and treatments. Arm yourself with knowledge that can help you make informed decisions about your health. The Strength of Determination and Positivity: A key part of overcoming any challenge is having a positive mindset. While it's normal to face setbacks or doubts, remember that each day presents an opportunity to grow and learn.

Your dedication to your well-being, whether through medical care, emotional strength, or personal growth, is a testament to your resilience and determination. Inspiring Stories of Change: People with epilepsy or other long-term conditions have transformed their lives by adapting, growing, and chasing their dreams. Their stories demonstrate that with perseverance and a positive attitude, one can overcome obstacles and reach their full potential.

Their stories show that obstacles can be hidden opportunities, teaching us patience, strength, and self-awareness. One final thought: remember, your diagnosis doesn't define you. Your journey is one-of-a-kind, filled with chances to discover, heal, and achieve. By embracing the process of personal growth and recognizing your inner potential, you unlock a life filled with purpose, meaning, and fulfillment. Whatever challenges come your way, trust in your resilience and the power of hope, because within you lies the strength to create a vibrant and meaningful future.

The Impact of Mindset and Dedication

Personal growth starts with building a strong and positive mindset - an inner foundation that influences how we see ourselves and the world. Our thoughts, beliefs, and attitude form an invisible roadmap for our actions and experiences. It's essential to understand that the universe doesn't rely on magic alone; it responds to the energy you put out through your thoughts, your body language, and your intentions.

When your mindset is aligned with clear and consistent action, it boosts your ability to drive meaningful change in your life. Many people underestimate the power of their mental attitude, but in reality, your belief system plays a crucial role in driving growth. A mindset grounded in hope, perseverance, and self-trust fosters resilience, allowing you to bounce back from setbacks and adapt to challenges.

When you face setbacks, don't see them as failures; see them as opportunities to learn and grow stronger. It's normal for progress to take time, and sometimes it's slow and gradual, especially when you're working on big goals or breaking old habits. That's why it's crucial to stay committed and keep pushing forward; it's what connects your goals to real results.

Every effort you make, no matter how small, lays the groundwork for future success. Acknowledge and celebrate these small wins; they demonstrate that your dedication is creating a ripple effect that will continue to grow over time. Your core beliefs and unshakeable determination serve as guiding forces, like the first explorers charting uncharted territories. They drive you beyond your comfort zone, helping you uncover strengths you never knew you had.

These qualities promote a mindset that views obstacles not as insurmountable barriers, but as chances to innovate and learn. Every small step paves the way for growth. Growth is a gradual process, often achieved through consistent, small steps. For instance, making a daily commitment, whether it's journaling, exercising, practicing mindfulness, or learning something new, gradually builds resilience and adaptability. These small actions add up, leading to significant transformations over time. They help you handle setbacks with poise, patience, and renewed focus.

When you face setbacks, remember that they're not the end, it's just part of the journey. Every obstacle presents an opportunity to refine your approach, strengthen your resolve, and deepen your self-awareness. You develop resilience not just through success, but also through persistence, pushing through tough times, learning from mistakes, and staying focused on your goal. Thrive, Don't Just Survive. This path to growth is about more than just getting by; it's about thriving.

It's about thriving in a proactive journey of building inner strength, discovering untapped abilities, and reaching your full potential. This path is more than just surviving; it's about flourishing by aligning your mindset with your actions and embracing each step with gratitude and courage. Along the way, you can unlock qualities and talents you may not have known you had. Remember, growth is a personal and ongoing process.

Achieving growth requires patience, self-compassion, and strong faith in your ability to improve. Even when progress is slow or setbacks happen again, keep the vision of who you're becoming in mind. Each effort, lesson, and challenge you face moves you closer to your best self. Trust that your dedication, regardless of how difficult things get, creates a solid base for future success.

Hold on to the faith that your perseverance is sowing seeds of change deep within you, and over time, these seeds will bloom into amazing, unexpected outcomes. Stay curious about your own potential. Foster a growth mindset that views failures as chances to learn. Acknowledge and celebrate your progress, no matter how small it may seem. By doing this, you reinforce your dedication to your journey, motivating yourself daily to become stronger, wiser, and more resilient.

At its core, personal development isn't about reaching a specific point; it's a lifelong journey powered by your inner strength, unwavering belief, and a dedication to becoming your most authentic self. Keep moving forward, and trust that the universe is working in your favor when your mindset aligns with your purpose. Your greatest achievements are waiting for you to claim them.

Insights Gained from Challenges

Some of the most valuable lessons I've learned in life and continue to learn every day have come from tough times, those moments that push us to our limits and test our strength. For people like me who live with epilepsy, each seizure, every moment of uncertainty, and each setback is a powerful teacher. These experiences may be uncomfortable and even scary, but they're opportunities to build resilience, gain a deeper understanding of ourselves, and see things from new angles.

Challenges aren't dead ends or signs of failure; they're chances for growth and change. When I face a tough time, I remind myself that "this too shall pass," a phrase that's rooted in patience and hope. It helps me stay calm and reminds me that pain or hardship are only temporary. Recognizing that tough feelings, although intense, won't last forever, allows me to stay present and composed, even in the midst of chaos.

Refining for Growth: One habit that has had a significant impact on me is setting aside time each week to reflect on recent challenges. This isn't just about listing setbacks, but about figuring out what I've learned from them. I ask myself key questions that help me focus on growth: What new insights have I gained from this experience? How has this challenge helped me grow personally? What strengths or qualities have I discovered or improved through this process? Writing down my thoughts, whether in a journal, recording voice memos, or taking digital notes, helps me stay focused on growth, possibilities, and resilience.

As I continue to practice, my outlook shifts from feeling overwhelmed or defeated to recognizing my ability to adapt and find strength. Here are some practical ways to get the most out of challenges: Take a Moment to Breathe: After a tough time, take a few deep breaths. Let yourself feel whatever emotions come up, fear, frustration, sadness, without judgment. This acknowledgment is essential for processing your experience in a constructive way. Reflect on Your Challenges: Use questions like the ones above to explore what each challenge has taught you about yourself, your values, or areas for growth.

Embrace Your Small Wins: Acknowledge the progress you've made, no matter how small it may seem. Maybe you stayed calm during a seizure or asked for help without hesitation. These small victories help build your confidence and resilience. Highlight Your Strengths: Consider qualities such as patience, courage, adaptability, or resourcefulness. Often, challenges reveal strengths you didn't know you had. Set Future Goals: Based on your reflections, set intentions for what's to come.

For example, you might focus on enhancing your stress management or building a more supportive network. The Power of a Growth Mindset: Having a growth mindset, which involves believing you can develop skills and understanding through effort, turns challenges into opportunities for growth. It helps you view setbacks as opportunities to learn and improve, guiding your personal growth. Every obstacle is an opportunity to discover new paths, build inner strength, and expand your perspective.

Embracing the Journey: A Call to Growth Remember, your journey is one of ongoing learning. Every challenge you face is a vital part of your story, showcasing your resilience and ability to bounce back. By reflecting on these experiences with openness and curiosity, you develop a mindset that welcomes growth, even in tough times. Stay the course with patience and faith, trusting that each challenge plays a role in your unfolding potential.

Today's insights set you up for even greater success tomorrow. The way you learn from tough times shows your real strength, the power to overcome, adapt, and become your best self. Try keeping a journal, setting time each week to reflect, and celebrating how you're growing stronger. As you learn from each experience, you're not just getting by; you're actively changing and becoming more resilient, more aware, and more confident in shaping your future with hope.

Cultivating gratitude.

Practicing gratitude is one of the most powerful ways to transform your perspective and enhance your overall well-being. It uniquely shifts your focus from what's missing or going wrong to recognizing the abundance already present in your life. When you make an effort to be grateful, it can significantly improve your mental health, emotional resilience, and even physical health. At its core, gratitude helps foster a mindset of abundance.

Instead of getting caught up in what you lack or haven't achieved, it invites you to appreciate and be grateful for the good things, lessons, and everyday joys that often get overlooked. This change in perspective doesn't mean giving up on your goals, but rather helps you develop a more balanced, contented, and joyful outlook. By focusing on where you are in this moment, you create space for greater happiness, peace, and a more open attitude towards new possibilities.

Why Gratitude Matters for a Better Lifestyle Practicing gratitude regularly has been shown to lower stress, reduce feelings of depression and anxiety, and improve sleep quality. It encourages positive emotions, which in turn strengthen your immune system and boost your energy. Plus, gratitude strengthens relationships by promoting kindness, empathy, and genuine connection, as you become more aware of the kindness others show you.

Practicing gratitude also helps build resilience a crucial trait for handling long-term health issues or life's unavoidable challenges. Focusing on the good, even in small ways, gives you the strength and motivation to push through tough times. To Incorporate Gratitude into Your Daily Routine, One easy way is to establish a daily gratitude practice.

Here are some practical suggestions: Pick a regular time each morning or evening that works for your schedule and use it to reflect on your thoughts. Consistency is key to making gratitude a habit. Keep a gratitude journal: write down three to five things you truly appreciate about your life. These might be something like a friend or family member's support, a recent accomplishment, a valuable lesson learned from a tough experience, or a beautiful sunset you enjoyed.

Get Specific and Genuine: Rather than saying something general like "I'm thankful for my family," try to pinpoint what about them or the support they gave that makes you grateful. For example, "I'm grateful for my sister's encouragement when I was having a tough week." Feel the Gratitude: As you write, take a moment to really let the appreciation sink in. Picture the moment, take a deep breath, and let yourself soak up the positive feelings that come up.

Being actively engaged with your emotions strengthens the impact of gratitude on your mindset. Try using visual reminders, such as a gratitude jar or sticky notes, to prompt reflection throughout the day, especially when things get busy or stressful. You can also express gratitude out loud, whether it's by journaling or telling someone you love how much you appreciate them. Even simple words of thanks can help strengthen your relationships and make you feel more grateful.

Developing a gratitude practice can have lasting benefits. By making gratitude a daily habit, you can change the way your brain works, focusing on the positive rather than the negative. This change can lead to a deeper sense of happiness, contentment, and satisfaction with life. Gratitude also helps build humility and perspective. When you appreciate the good things in your life, you understand that many of them aren't just the result of your own hard work, but also luck, kindness from others, and other factors outside your control.

This helps you feel more connected and grateful for the bigger picture in life. To start, focus on small things. Even on tough days, try to find something to be thankful for - maybe it's just taking a deep breath or enjoying a cup of tea. As you keep practicing, this habit will become second nature, changing your attitude to be more positive and open.

Remember that practicing gratitude isn't about ignoring hardships or pretending everything is perfect. It's about intentionally recognizing life's blessings along with its challenges and developing a balanced, resilient outlook filled with optimism. This mindset attracts more abundance and joy into your life, encouraging a lifestyle rooted in appreciation and hope. By incorporating gratitude into your daily routine, you'll gradually see positive changes in your experiences, relationships, and inner self, leading to a more fulfilling, peaceful, and vibrant way of living.

Self-Discovery Activities

Self-awareness is a key part of personal growth; it's like a compass that points you in the direction of fulfillment and authenticity. Setting aside time to regularly reflect on your thoughts, feelings, and actions helps you determine which practices are beneficial for you and which areas require more attention or adjustment. This ongoing process brings clarity and purpose to your journey, ensuring your actions align with your core goals and values.

Embracing the Power of Self-Reflection: Taking time for honest self-reflection lets you step away from the chaos of daily life and examine your inner thoughts. It's a chance to evaluate your progress, recognize achievements, and face areas that need improvement. By doing so, you gain a deeper understanding of the patterns, habits, and beliefs that shape your decisions and emotions. Building a Self-Reflection Habit. One way to nurture self-awareness is to keep a regular self-reflection journal.

Don't worry about making it formal or lengthy - just be consistent and genuine. Writing down your experiences, feelings, and observations regularly helps you better understand yourself and see your growth over time. To get started, try exploring these meaningful questions in your journal: What strengths am I proud of right now or relying on? What areas of my life or myself need more attention or care? What goals or values are currently driving me? What challenges or setbacks have I faced recently, and how did I deal with them? What habits or beliefs might be holding me back? What small wins or accomplishments have I achieved that I might have missed? Be Honest and Kind to Yourself. It's crucial to approach this exercise with honesty and self-compassion.

Try not to be too hard on yourself; instead, view your reflections as an opportunity to learn and grow. If you spot areas that need work, view them as chances to learn, not as failures. Take time each month to review your journal entries and identify what's working and what's not. Approach your reflections with an open mind: What patterns or insights keep popping up? Have you become stronger in certain areas? Are there habits or thought processes that need to change? How have your goals and motivations shifted? Use this review time to recognize your progress and accomplishments.

Recognizing small victories boosts motivation and helps lock in positive habits. On the other hand, if you notice areas where progress has stalled, consider adjusting your approach. For instance, if a specific goal feels too big, break it down into smaller, more manageable steps. If doubts or fears persist, seek practical ways to build confidence or find additional support. Try Out Practical Activities Beyond Just Journaling. You can take your self-discovery to the next level with activities like Meditation or mindfulness practices. These focused exercises help you observe your thoughts and feelings without judgment.

Visualization: Envisioning your ideal self or future helps clarify your goals. Creating a "Values List" outlines core principles that guide your decisions, serving as a guiding star on your journey. Feedback Seeking: Asking trusted friends, mentors, or coaches for honest feedback on your strengths and areas for growth. The Long-Term Impact: Regularly practicing self-reflection and honest assessment fosters self-trust, enables you to adapt to changing circumstances, and aligns your actions with your evolving goals.

It helps you build resilience by increasing your awareness of your ability to handle tough situations and learn from them. Remember, self-discovery is a journey that never ends. There's no finish line. Every new insight, breakthrough, and change is a step toward a deeper understanding of yourself and a more fulfilling life. Be kind to yourself, appreciate your progress, and stay committed to becoming the best version of yourself. With consistent self-awareness, you can make intentional choices, live with purpose, and create a life that truly reflects your authentic self.

Cultivating Developmental Habits

Forming habits that encourage lifelong growth, foster gratitude, and increase self-awareness are crucial to a happy and resilient life. When you make these practices a part of your daily routine, they lay the groundwork for ongoing personal development and lasting change. Developing these habits isn't about being perfect, but about putting in consistent effort and being intentional.

Here's a thorough plan for incorporating effective, growth-driven habits into your daily routine:

1. Consistency: The Key to Building Habits. Set aside a few minutes each day, whether in the morning, at lunch, or before bed, to engage in activities such as practicing gratitude, journaling, or visualization. Consistency builds momentum; even small daily efforts accumulate and lead to significant change over time.

For example, try writing down three things you're grateful for, whether it's a major achievement or a small act of kindness. Another idea is to reflect on your feelings, what you've learned, or your personal goals. This practice helps clear your mind and strengthens your resolve to grow.

Visualization: Take a few moments to vividly picture your ideal self or a goal you want to achieve, becoming emotionally invested as if it were already a reality. The goal isn't to be perfect every day, but to consistently show up and build discipline and dedication.

2. Patience: Embracing Slow and Steady Progress. Big changes take time. It's important to recognize that progress can be slow and unpredictable. Develop patience by trusting the process and understanding that growth involves setbacks, small wins, and valuable lessons learned along the way. Remember: Every effort matters, no matter how small it seems at the moment. Mistakes and delays are all part of the learning journey.

They offer valuable feedback that helps you refine your approach and build stronger resilience. As you make progress, it adds up over time. By focusing on daily habits, you can gradually transform your mindset and life.

3. Surround Yourself with a Supportive Network. A positive environment can significantly accelerate personal growth. Make an effort to surround yourself with people who motivate, support, and lift you up. Look for mentors, friends who support you, or community groups that share your values and goals.

Fill your time with inspiring content: listen to motivational podcasts, read uplifting books, or follow social media accounts that focus on positivity and growth. Make a space for self-reflection: designate a quiet spot in your home or workspace for journaling or meditation, where you can focus without distractions. Surrounding yourself with a supportive environment boosts your motivation, gives you a sense of accountability, and helps you stay committed even when things get tough.

4. Celebrate Small Wins: Acknowledge and honor every step forward, no matter how minor. Celebrating achievements boosts your confidence and reinforces positive habits. For example: Finishing a week of daily gratitude journaling, overcoming a fear, trying something new, or making progress on a personal or professional goal. Recognizing your efforts fuels motivation and builds momentum for continued growth.

5. Perseverance and Commitment: Recognize that perseverance is key, particularly when progress feels slow or challenges come up. Building a growth mindset requires unwavering commitment and a conviction that steady effort will ultimately yield results. Push through setbacks: Treat them as chances to learn and adjust.

Remain committed: Reiterate the reasons for your initial motivation and maintain focus on your long-term objectives. Adapt as necessary: Demonstrating flexibility in your methodology enables you to identify what functions most effectively for you without diminishing your progress.

1. Daily Practice Example: Morning Affirmations and Reflection. A practical way to strengthen your habits is to begin each day with positive affirmations and gratitude. For instance, you might say: "I'm capable of growth," "Today, I'll focus on learning," or "I deserve success and happiness."

Take a moment to reflect on what you're grateful for, setting a positive tone for the day. Also, spend a few minutes thinking about what you've learned recently, whether from the previous day or week. Ask yourself: What have I learned about myself lately? What areas do I need to work on or focus on? What small success can I celebrate today? As you make these practices a regular part of your routine, they'll become second nature, providing you with steady clarity and purpose in your personal growth.

In summary, developing these habits is a lifelong process that requires patience, consistency, and kindness. By committing just a few minutes each day, building a supportive environment, recognizing small victories, and staying committed, you lay the groundwork for genuine, lasting growth. Put these habits into practice.

Final Reflections on Development and Opportunity

As you navigate this journey, you'll see that embracing a mindset based on abundance and self-trust can bring about profound changes. When you tap into your limitless potential, you unlock doors to opportunities that stretch beyond your current understanding, recognizing that your capacity for growth far surpasses what you once thought possible, despite any external limitations.

Viewing challenges as opportunities for growth, rather than impossible hurdles, builds resilience and a commitment to learning. Every tough situation teaches you something about your strengths, weaknesses, and where you need to improve. Cultivating gratitude along the way helps you focus on the good things, leading to a sense of satisfaction and motivation, even when things don't go as planned.

Self-discovery is a lifelong journey, a constantly changing process of understanding who you are, what you care about, and what you aim to achieve. By staying curious, being honest with yourself, and embracing growth at every turn, you can make the most of life's chances to grow and be fulfilled. Remember, by cultivating this mindset and welcoming life's lessons with an open heart and gratitude, you give yourself the power to reach your full potential and create a life that's truly meaningful and abundant one step, one lesson, and one discovery at a time.

Conclusion

Personal growth is a continuous path, not a one-time achievement. Gratitude sets the stage for abundance, teaching you to appreciate what you have while paving the way for new opportunities. Self-awareness serves as your guiding light, offering clarity and direction as you explore your true passions and purpose. By acknowledging your aspirations and taking intentional action today, you lay the groundwork for reaching your potential. Developing habits that nurture both your mind and spirit, like daily reflection, gratitude practices, and ongoing learning, reveals extraordinary possibilities within you. Remember, the life you envision isn't just a far-off dream; it's a reality within reach, waiting for you to step into it. Today marks the start of that journey. Embrace personal growth, gratitude, and self-discovery as daily essentials. Face challenges with confidence and illuminate your path with unwavering clarity and purpose. Your brighter future begins now.

Welcome to Action.

Have faith in your abilities and know you have the strength and resilience to overcome any challenge. Seeing obstacles as opportunities to learn and grow changes your mindset from one of fear to one of empowerment. Keep in mind, setbacks are just part of the process; each one teaches you something valuable that brings you closer to your goals. The life you envision isn't just a far-off dream; it's an achievable reality that starts with small, intentional steps.

Every action counts, no matter how small, and paves the way for real change. Taking that first step today and making a consistent effort sets you on the path to greatness. As you move forward, stay positive and focused on your goals both physically and mentally. Don't get caught up in immediate doubts or fears; look ahead to your purpose.

Walk with confidence, knowing your perseverance and dedication are your biggest strengths. The world is full of possibilities and opportunities, just waiting for your unique talents; all you need is the drive to pursue them. Start your journey now. Take that first step today, and trust that every effort, no matter how small, brings you closer to the life of fulfillment and success you want. Your path to greatness starts right here.

Chapter 11:
Tools for Self-Discovery and Personal Growth

Starting on the path of self-discovery and personal growth is more than just trying to be a "better" version of yourself. It's a profound and life-changing journey to tap into your true self, the core of who you are beyond your roles, expectations, and outside influences. At your core, you're already whole, worthy, and vibrant, with a natural ability to create a life that reflects your deepest desires and values.

However, in the chaos of everyday life, stress, societal pressures, doubts, and distractions can cause your authentic self to get lost or forgotten. The constant pull of responsibilities, routines, and habits can detach you from what's truly real. That's why it's essential to make space for self-awareness and reflection on purpose. This chapter offers a comprehensive toolkit to help you reconnect with your true self.

These practical tools and purposeful strategies act as your trusted guides, helping you reveal the layers of doubt, fear, or superficiality that often cloud your vision. The goal isn't perfection, but progress, building self-awareness step by step, day by day. Practical Tools for Self-Discovery and Growth: Mindfulness and Meditation: Make it a habit to regularly practice techniques that keep your attention focused on the present moment.

These routines help calm your mind, cut down on distractions, and bring clarity to your true thoughts and feelings. Journaling is a great way to start: set aside a few minutes each day or week to write about your experiences, emotions, and thoughts. This process helps you see patterns that repeat, gain a deeper understanding of yourself, and clarify what truly matters to you.

Reflective Practices: Make a habit of asking yourself thought-provoking questions, such as: Who am I beyond my job titles? What really matters to me? What are my most profound aspirations? Reflecting on these questions helps you tap into your authentic self. Clarifying your Purpose and Values: Identify what truly matters to you in life, your principles, passions, and goals. Knowing your core values serves as a guiding light, aligning your decisions with your inner truth.

Visualization and Affirmations: Use visualization techniques to imagine your ideal life and employ affirmations to cultivate self-worth and confidence. These mental exercises can significantly boost motivation and self-belief. Physical Movement and Self-Care: Engage in activities like yoga or walking that connect your mind and body, helping you tune into your physical and emotional needs. Feedback and Support: Seek honest feedback from friends, mentors, or coaches who can provide a fresh perspective and encouragement.

At times, outside perspectives can shed light on aspects of yourself that you might miss. Build Rituals for Connection: Establish personal habits, such as morning reflections, gratitude practices, or evening check-ins, that strengthen your dedication to self-awareness and growth. Intentional Use of Strategies: Becoming authentic requires deliberate effort.

Regularly setting aside time for reflection, keeping an open mind, and being gentle with yourself during setbacks are essential. Remember, growth is a slow process that occurs through small, steady steps. This toolkit is designed not only to guide you when you're feeling lost or uncertain but also to help you make self-discovery a natural part of your daily routine.

As you work with these tools over time, they help you uncover the layers that block your inner truth, revealing a more vibrant, aligned, and empowered version of yourself. In brief, this chapter offers practical and realistic tools to help you reconnect with your authentic self. By incorporating these strategies into your daily life, you'll create a path to genuine self-awareness, aligned living, and long-term personal growth. Your authentic self is waiting. These tools will help you uncover it, one step at a time.

Mindfulness and Meditation Practices: Cultivating Present Awareness

Self-reflection starts with a firm commitment to being fully present in the moment. Mindfulness practice is about developing a non-judgmental awareness of your thoughts, feelings, and physical sensations, accepting whatever comes up without trying to push it away, avoid it, or break it down. This acceptance creates a safe space where you can observe your internal thoughts, triggers, fears, and aspirations objectively.

When you engage with your inner experiences with compassion and curiosity, you cultivate a deeper understanding of your habitual reactions and thought patterns. This increased awareness enables you to pause prior to responding impulsively, thereby empowering you to select thoughtful and deliberate responses rather than defaulting to habitual, often unproductive reactions. Over time, this practice promotes emotional regulation, mitigates stress, and nurtures inner tranquility.

Practical Exercises for Cultivating Mindfulness

1. Two-Minute Grounding Exercise: This straightforward yet efficacious practice facilitates anchoring oneself in the present moment, particularly during instances of elevated stress or distraction. Find a comfortable and quiet environment where you may sit or stand still. Gently close your eyes, should you feel comfortable doing so. Take a deep inhalation through the nose, fully expanding your lungs. Sustain the breath for approximately four seconds, perceiving the sensation of expansion in your chest and abdomen.

Exhale deliberately and consistently over a duration of six seconds, paying meticulous attention to the sensations associated with the act of releasing air and experiencing relaxation. Concentrate your attention exclusively on the physical sensations related to your respiration, specifically, how the air feels as it enters and exits your nostrils, as well as the rise and fall of your chest or abdomen. Should your mind begin to stray, kindly acknowledge the distraction without criticism and calmly redirect your focus back to your breath.

Use this grounding technique as often as needed. It's a great way to get a quick reset or clear your head whenever you need it.

1. Body Scan Meditation This practice fosters profound relaxation and develops an enhanced awareness of bodily sensations, thereby considerably alleviating stress and fostering present-moment consciousness: Lie in a comfortable position on your back, whether on a bed or a yoga mat. Keep your arms relaxed at your sides and ensure your legs are uncrossed. Gently close

your eyes and take several deep breaths to anchor yourself in the present moment. Commence by directing your attention towards your toes.

Notice sensations like warmth, coolness, tingling, or tension. Slowly move your attention upward through your feet, ankles, calves, knees, thighs, and other areas, observing each without trying to change anything. As you focus on each part, imagine releasing tension as you exhale or as you relax. Spend a few moments on each area before moving up through your body, ending at your face and head.

As you go through the process, stay gentle and non-judgmental with any discomfort or distracting thoughts. Just acknowledge them and refocus on the body part you're currently scanning. This exercise helps build body awareness, reduces stress, and gives you a sense of calm. For those just starting out or looking for guidance, mobile apps like Insight Timer, Headspace, or Calm provide easy-to-follow, guided sessions that can fit into your daily routine.

These platforms offer a diverse range of meditation techniques and durations from brief two-minute exercises to more extended, immersive sessions, thereby making mindfulness accessible to individuals regardless of their schedules. Cultivating Mindfulness as a Daily Routine. The fundamental aspect of deriving benefits from mindfulness practices is consistency and patience. It is advisable to dedicate a few minutes each day, perhaps in the morning to establish a tranquil tone, or in the evening to relax. Over time, these moments of present awareness can become inherent, effortless components of daily life, enabling individuals to approach each moment with clarity, patience, and compassion.

Final Thoughts: Keep in mind that mindfulness isn't about reaching perfection or clearing your mind completely. It's about developing a kind and accepting awareness of what's happening in the present, regardless of its form. Through regular practice, you'll gain a deeper understanding of yourself, enhance your emotional control, and experience greater peace of mind. These skills help you live more fully, making each moment more valuable and less overwhelming. Start today your path to mindfulness and inner calm is within your grasp, one breath and one moment at a time.

Journaling Prompts: Uncover Your Authentic Self

Journaling is more than just documenting your daily events; it's a powerful tool for gaining self-awareness, understanding your emotions, organizing your thoughts, and ultimately creating the life you want. Regular writing allows you to tap into your true self without fear of judgment or self-censorship. When you sit down to write, you create a safe space for your inner thoughts and feelings to emerge naturally.

As time passes, this practice helps uncover patterns, clarify your values, and highlight aspects of yourself that may have gone unnoticed. Simply writing down or typing out your thoughts can trigger breakthroughs, foster growth, and reinforce your commitment to authenticity. Here are some thoughtfully created prompts to incorporate into your daily journaling, helping you explore your inner self more deeply: What new insights have I gained about my personal growth today? Think about what you've learned about yourself, new strengths, challenges, or perspectives, and how these insights influence your journey.

What emotion am I pushing away, and what's behind this avoidance? Face feelings that might be tough or bottled up, like fear, sadness, or anger. Think about why these emotions are hard to confront and explore ways to gently work through them. How do I see my perfect life unfolding over the next three years? Let your imagination run wild, think about your relationships, career, health, passions, and personal growth. Use this vision to motivate your daily actions that align with your goals.

What would I do if I knew I'd succeed? Picture a future where all obstacles are gone. What big goals would you chase? This question helps you figure out what you really want and overcome self-doubt. Which part of me needs love and care right now? Identify areas of yourself that need kindness, such as your body, mind, or spirit, and consider simple ways to nurture them.

Effective Journaling: A Step-by-Step Guide. Set aside 5-10 minutes each day to write freely. Use a timer to stay focused and promote non-judgmental expression, avoiding overthinking or self-censorship. Consistency is essential; whether you write in the morning, during lunch, or before bed, making journaling a daily habit helps you build ongoing self-awareness.

What matters most is that you write, not what you write about. Regularly reflecting on your thoughts and feelings builds a strong sense of authenticity and self-awareness. Don't worry about perfecting your grammar, spelling, or structure; just let your thoughts flow freely. Be kind to yourself, especially when navigating tough emotions or confronting difficult truths. The goal is to cultivate a gentle and curious connection with your inner world. To take your practice to the next level, try these additional tips: Create a cozy environment by finding a quiet spot where you feel at ease and undisturbed.

Consider playing soft music, which is what I usually do when I am writing or relaxing with a cup of tea nearby, to make your practice more inviting. Use a dedicated journal or digital application: Having a special journal or application reserved for self-reflection enhances the intentionality and significance of the experience. Reflect on your journaling experience periodically: Every few weeks, review your entries to observe patterns, monitor growth, or identify recurring themes worth exploring further. Be patient and persistent: Self-awareness develops gradually. Celebrate small insights, and trust that consistency will deepen your understanding of yourself over time.

Remember: Journaling is a personal journey a revealing, nurturing, and empowering practice. By dedicating only a few minutes each day, you establish a valuable tool for continuous self-discovery, authenticity, and transformation. Embrace this invaluable time to listen profoundly to your inner voice and to articulate your evolving narrative.

Visualization Methods: Imagining Success

Visualization is a powerful tool that can boost your confidence, motivation, and focus. By vividly imagining achieving your goals or living your ideal life, your brain treats those images as if they were real experiences. This mental rehearsal gives you energy, strengthens your conviction, and drives the actions needed to turn your vision into reality. Studies have found that using all your senses in visualization makes the experience more engaging and effective.

When your mental images are rich and vivid, your subconscious mind receives a compelling message that success is not merely possible but assured. Here is the methodology for effective visualization.

1. Set a Clear Intention Start by defining your goal or the vision you want to bring into reality. For instance, imagine living a balanced life, reaching a career milestone, or building strong, meaningful relationships. Be clear about what you want to achieve.

2. Imagine Your Ideal Day in Five Years. Take a moment to find a peaceful spot where you can unwind without distractions. Close your eyes and take a few slow, calming breaths to calm your mind. Now, picture your life five years from now and try to visualize it as clearly as possible: Where will you be? Envision your surroundings, your home, office, or environment. What do you see, feel, and hear? Who's with you? Picture your loved ones, friends, or colleagues, and imagine their expressions, gestures, and voices.

What's your ideal day look like? Picture yourself pursuing a passion project, enjoying your hobbies, or unwinding in nature. What emotions are you feeling most strongly? Feel the joy, pride, gratitude, or calmness that comes with living this dream life.

Use all your senses: Sight: Take in the vibrant colors, lighting, and details. Sound: Pay attention to the sounds around you, laughter, music, nature, or ambient noise.

Touch: Feel the softness of fabrics, the warmth of sunlight, or the gentle breeze on your skin. Smell: Take in the aroma of familiar or uplifting scents, like flowers, food, or fresh air.

Taste: Imagine the flavors that define your ideal day, such as a favorite meal or drink. Allow yourself to immerse in this scene for five to ten minutes, letting the vividness and emotions settle in.

3. Make Visualization a Habit. Consistency is essential. Aim to visualize daily, ideally in the morning to start your day or before bed to reinforce your goals. The more you repeat this process, the stronger your conviction grows, transforming vague aspirations into powerful motivations for action. Why Visualization Works When you visualize

success consistently, your brain develops neural pathways aligned with your goals, making it easier to take action.

Visualization can increase your confidence, ease anxiety, and help you overcome doubts or fears. As you practice, your subconscious begins to look for opportunities and solutions that support your goals, guiding you toward actions and decisions that align with your ideal future. To get the most out of your visualization practice, try these practical tips: Find a quiet, comfortable spot where you can reduce distractions and set aside time to relax and focus on your visualization.

Keep a journal or record yourself: Write down your vision or record it in your own voice to solidify your commitment.

Use affirmations: Combine visualization with positive statements, such as "I'm capable," "I deserve success," or "I'm taking steps daily toward my dreams."

Visualize with feeling: Connect emotionally with your scene, feel the joy or gratitude as if your vision is already happening. This strengthens your belief and motivation. Follow with action: After each session, pick one small step you can take today to move closer to your vision.

One last thing to remember: visualization is more than just daydreaming - it's a proactive tool that aligns your mind, emotions, and actions with your desired future. By engaging all your senses and practicing regularly, you'll develop stronger conviction, spark motivation, and create momentum for real change. Take that first step today and see how your vivid imagination sets the stage for remarkable accomplishments.

Affirmations and Positive Self-Talk: Empower Yourself Through Your Words

What you say to yourself has a big impact on your outside experiences. The way you talk to yourself, whether with kindness or criticism, directly affects your confidence, mindset, and overall well-being. Constant self-criticism can harm your self-esteem, create obstacles to success, and foster a fear of failure. On the other hand, being intentional and kind to yourself can help you grow, be more resilient, and have a mindset that attracts good things.

Practicing daily affirmations involves intentionally choosing empowering statements that emphasize your strengths, values, and potential. These affirmations serve as gentle reminders that you're worthy, capable, and deserving of success, happiness, and love. Repeating them regularly can gradually reprogram your subconscious mind to foster a mindset focused on growth and abundance. The power of daily affirmations strengthens your core beliefs: carefully selected affirmations help solidify your sense of self in strength and possibility.

Pushes back against negative thoughts: They act as a counter to self-doubt, anxiety, and self-sabotage. Boosts confidence: Repeating affirmations can increase your self-esteem, making it easier to tackle challenges head-on. Draws in positivity: When paired with genuine emotion, affirmations can change your perspective and lead you to new opportunities.

Sample affirmations for daily practice: I am transforming into the person I am meant to be. I possess confidence in my capacity to make sound decisions. I am deserving of love, happiness, and abundance. I hold the qualities I presently possess, and I am developing each day. I focus on cultivating thoughts that foster my growth. I am resilient and capable of overcoming any obstacle. I am worthy of success and tranquility. Every day, I am making progress toward my objectives.

Practical Strategies for Incorporating Affirmations Speak aloud daily: Dedicate a few moments each morning or evening to speak your affirmations aloud. The physical act of vocalization reinforces belief more powerfully than silent repetition. Practice in front of a mirror: Stand in front of a mirror, meet your own gaze, and repeat your affirmations.

Practicing affirmations can boost your self-awareness, sincerity, and confidence. Use them in tough moments: When doubt, fear, or negative thoughts creep in, take a moment to remind yourself of your affirmations. Swap anxiety for empowering statements. Keep them top of mind: Write your affirmations down and place them somewhere you'll see them often, such as on your mirror, computer, or fridge, to stay positive throughout the day. Make them a habit: Incorporate affirmations into your daily routine, whether it's during your commute, workout, or before bed, to make them a natural part of your thinking.

Additional Tips for Powerful Self-Talk Be specific and genuine: Tailor affirmations to your personal goals and feelings. Authenticity makes them more effective. Use the present tense: State affirmations as if they are already true, like "I am confident," not "I will be confident." Connect with your emotions: Feel the truth of your affirmations and imagine what it's like to embody those qualities or achieve those goals.

Avoid negative phrasing: Focus on what you wish to affirm about yourself, rather than what you seek to avoid. Instead of "I am not anxious," consider stating "I am calm and centered." The long-term impact of consistent practice with affirmations and positive self-talk involves gradually reconfiguring your internal dialogue, thereby replacing limiting beliefs with empowering ones. This transformation in mindset improves your perspective, increases resilience, and attracts more positive circumstances into your life.

Remember, your words spoken with conviction possess the capacity to transform your inner world and, ultimately, your external reality. Initiate this process today. Select affirmations that resonate profoundly with you, articulate them aloud with sincerity and emotion, and allow your words to serve as the foundation for a more confident, resilient, and optimistic self. Your mindset shapes your reality. Foster one characterized by empowerment, love, and boundless potential.

Set Achievable Goals by Leaning on Your Strengths

Personal growth usually happens through small, intentional steps, not huge leaps. Setting clear, achievable goals keeps you motivated and helps build confidence as you move forward. The SMART framework is a great way to set goals, making them Specific, Measurable, Achievable, Relevant, and Time-bound.

Specific: Clearly define your objectives to ensure clarity in your goals. Ambiguous ambitions such as "get fit" are less effective than well-defined targets. Instead, specify, "I will walk for 20 minutes, three times a week." Measurable: Establish your methods for monitoring progress. Will you track your walks via a calendar or using a fitness application? Setting quantifiable milestones guarantees that you can effectively observe your development.

Take a realistic approach by honestly assessing what is feasible given your current circumstances. Setting goals that are too ambitious can lead to frustration, while challenging yet achievable objectives can encourage ongoing effort and motivation. Make sure your goals are relevant by aligning them with your core values and long-term vision. For example, if health is a priority, starting with simple physical activities can enhance your overall well-being. Additionally, include a deadline in your goals to create a sense of urgency and purpose. For instance, commit to a walking routine for the next 30 days to stay accountable and reflect on your progress.

For example, instead of saying something vague like "I want to be healthier," set a specific goal, such as "I'll walk briskly for 20 minutes, three times a week, for the next month." This targeted approach helps you stay consistent and makes progress more tangible. Celebrate Your Milestones: Recognize and celebrate every achievement, no matter how small. Finishing your first week of regular walks or sticking to your schedule for a month is worth acknowledging. Celebrating your accomplishments boosts your confidence, reinforces positive habits, and motivates you to keep improving. Keeping a journal or a success log can help remind you of how far you've come, which is especially helpful during slow periods or setbacks.

Embrace Your Complete Self: Illuminate Without Regret. Recognizing your intrinsic worth is crucial for personal growth and development. Self-love is not merely a comforting expression; it involves respecting your needs, establishing healthy boundaries, forgiving yourself for past mistakes, and remaining receptive to future opportunities. It is about nurturing one's inner environment, free from dependence on external validation or approval.

Take Care of Your Needs: Make time to determine what truly nourishes your body, mind, and spirit. Whether it's rest, alone time, social connections, or creative outlets, prioritize those needs without feeling guilty. Set Healthy Boundaries: Guard your energy by setting limits with others and yourself. Saying no to things that drain or distract you is a sign of self-respect.

Practice self-forgiveness by releasing past mistakes and recognizing that growth involves trial, error, and learning. Forgive yourself as a key part of your ongoing development. Stay open to future opportunities by keeping an open heart for new experiences, growth avenues, and relationships. Understand that your potential is limitless, and the future offers many possibilities.

Everyone is Special. Your unique qualities, talents, and viewpoints are all precious. You're one-of-a-kind, and the world needs your presence. By approaching yourself with kindness and confidence, you'll let your genuine light shine through.

Motivational Reminder: The primary obstacle you encounter is frequently internal, comprising doubts, fears, or limiting beliefs. Overcoming these internal barriers constitutes the initial step toward liberation. Recognize that you are already complete and capable; self-acceptance is essential to unlocking your full potential. Final Reflection: Embrace your wholeness with pride. Have confidence that your journey is precisely where it should be. Celebrate your uniqueness, nurture your needs, and radiate confidently because the world genuinely benefits from your brilliance.

Chapter 12:
Envisioning What Lies Ahead: My Continuing Journey

Most of us have dreams of living a life with purpose, vitality, and genuine fulfillment, dreams that extend beyond merely getting by or following the same routine. These hopes can be big goals, such as starting a career that matters or forming strong connections, or they can be more subtle desires, like finding inner peace or pursuing a lifelong passion. Each of these desires is special and unique, revealing different parts of who we truly are.

However, amidst the pursuit of these aspirations, a vital question arises: Are these aspirations genuinely aligned with our fundamental purpose, or are they merely transient desires or societal expectations? Recognizing the distinction is essential because substantive change and development originate from intentions anchored in our authentic values, rather than external influences or superficial cravings. This chapter encourages reflection on one's personal transformation journey. It underscores that change is seldom linear; it encompasses overcoming fears, challenging comfort zones, and managing setbacks.

Still, within these challenges, there's great potential for growth and discovery, allowing you to learn more about yourself, build resilience, and gain a deeper understanding of who you truly are and what you truly want out of life. Reflecting Realistically on the Path to Change: Acknowledge the Challenges: Personal growth often involves discomfort. Whether you're facing fears of failure, confronting limiting beliefs, or making tough decisions, these obstacles can seem overwhelming. But they're crucial stepping stones toward reaching your full potential.

Embracing the Process: Change is not something that can be hurried; it is a gradual and unfolding journey. Throughout this journey, it is necessary to exercise patience, persistence, and self-compassion. When setbacks occur, they should be regarded as opportunities for learning rather than obstacles.

Celebrate Small Wins: Every step forward, no matter how small, counts as progress. Recognizing these achievements builds confidence and motivates ongoing growth.

Staying True to Your Purpose: Make it a point to regularly reflect on whether your actions align with your core values and goals. This helps keep your journey authentic and fulfilling.

Practical Perspectives for Moving Forward: Set Intentional Goals - Identify goals that align with your values and passions, and let them serve as your guiding light. These goals will point you in a direction that matters and give you a sense of purpose.

Take time to reflect and be mindful. Regular check-ins with yourself can help you discover what you're learning, what excites you, or what fears you need to face. By being aware of these things, you can make sure your efforts stay on track with your purpose.

Stay Flexible: Embrace the idea that your goals may shift as you grow. What matters most today might change, and that's a natural part of personal growth.

Find Support and Inspiration: Surround yourself with people who bring out the best in you, such as mentors, friends, or groups that inspire and encourage you to grow in a genuine way.

Building a Future that's Truly Fulfilled

Every journey is one-of-a-kind, a path woven with your own hopes, challenges, setbacks, and successes. The road may be bumpy, but each step brings you closer to understanding who you are and what you're meant to do. By embracing this process with openness and patience, you'll create a life where your actions match your inner values.

Remember, the future is not merely a subject for dreaming; it is an advancing reality that you actively shape through each decision, effort, and act of courage. Your aspirations serve as the seeds of potential. Cultivate them with careful consideration, welcome the challenges associated with growth, and have confidence that your genuine purpose awaits patiently to be uncovered and realized. Your ongoing journey of transformation is dynamic, vibrant, and filled with boundless possibilities.

Second Chance for Positive Change

After facing many challenges before my brain surgery, life felt like a dull routine, days merging into one another, filled with daily habits and minor distractions that left me feeling disconnected from my true goals. It felt like I was just getting by, stuck in a cycle of limitations and repeated struggles that wore me down and blurred my vision for the future.

When I finally had the surgery, it was like getting a second chance, a chance to start fresh, not just with my physical health, but with my mindset and my whole outlook on life. That moment was a turning point for me, a new beginning that sparked a renewed passion. It was as if I was starting a new chapter, one filled with the potential for growth and change that I'd once thought was impossible.

For me, this procedure was more than just a medical necessity; it was a turning point, a spark that ignited a profound inner transformation and revealed new insights and priorities. As I recovered physically, I noticed a significant shift in my mindset. Before, I had seen my circumstances through the lens of limitations and setbacks. But now, I started to view the world in a different light: not as a series of impossible obstacles, but as a vast canvas waiting for me to bring my creative energy and intentional action to it.

This awakening sparked a string of thought-provoking questions: What if this is my one shot at building the life I've always dreamed of? What if I took this second chance to welcome change, chase my passions, and live by my true values? This change in perspective was life-changing, motivating me to tackle life with purpose, hope, and intentional action.

That moment marked the start of a deliberate journey toward personal growth. I came to understand the value of making intentional choices, taking small steps every day toward my goals, rather than waiting for the perfect moment or external circumstances to change. It drove home the importance of mindset and the significant impact of believing in the potential for renewal, regardless of the setbacks or limitations I'd faced.

This experience has reinforced the idea that life can sometimes provide pivotal moments, second chances that spark crucial change.

It's a reminder that even in tough times, our circumstances can be the starting point for a more genuine, vibrant, and fulfilling life. With a fresh perspective and determination, I now see my life as a blank canvas, waiting for me to paint it with purpose and resilience. This second chance is a gift, a chance to create a new path and become the person I'm truly meant to be.

Take Charge: Empowering Strategies for Action

Turning your dreams into reality takes more than just wanting something or having a positive attitude; it demands intentional, purposeful action. The sheer size of a big goal can often leave you feeling overwhelmed or hesitant, making it tempting to put it off or give up altogether. But breaking down these bigger visions into smaller, achievable steps makes the path to your aspirations not only possible but also inspiring.

Here's a hands-on guide to help you turn your intentions into action, giving you the power to drive your own growth and success.

1. Turning Your Dreams into Reality Vague hopes and abstract aspirations can easily fade or feel out of reach. To bring your vision to life, try writing down your goals in concrete, specific terms. Instead of saying "I want to be healthier," say "I want to lose 10 pounds and improve my fitness by walking 20 minutes a day." Use vivid imagery and descriptive language to create a clear picture of your ideal outcome, which helps you set a clear direction. Create a visual board, journal, or digital document to keep your goals top of mind and motivate you. By writing down your goals, you turn them into actionable plans, creating a personal roadmap that clarifies your purpose and keeps you accountable.

2. Break Down Your Goals Once you've clarified your goals, break them into smaller, concrete tasks. Ask yourself: What can I do this week to move closer to my goal? Examples include: researching resources, tutorials, or local classes related to your goal; reaching out to a mentor, coach, or someone you admire for guidance; creating a mini-strategy or plan outlining the steps; setting mini-deadlines for each task to stay

focused; gathering necessary materials; or scheduling dedicated time on your calendar.

1. Focus on First Steps, Not Perfection. Getting caught up in perfectionism and fearing failure can hinder your progress. Instead, adopt a mindset of starting where you are, with what you have. Acknowledge that your current resources, time, skills, or knowledge are enough to get started.

Your first step could be as simple as sending an email, making a phone call, or dedicating 10 minutes to your project today. Remember, progress often comes from steady effort, not perfection. Small, imperfect actions add up over time, ultimately leading to big change. Steer clear of waiting for the perfect moment; real growth happens right now.

Extra Tips for Taking Action:

Set Priorities: Focus on just a few key actions each week, rather than trying to do too much. This helps build momentum and keeps you focused on what's most important.

Keep Track of Your Progress: Use a notebook, checklist, or app to stay on top of the steps you've finished. Recognizing your accomplishments can be a big motivator.

Review and Adjust: Take the time to reassess your plan regularly and ensure it continues to serve you well. If something feels too tough or not crucial, make changes. Being flexible is essential for achieving lasting progress.

Establish a Routine: Develop daily or weekly habits, such as planning your next step on Sundays or reviewing your goals each morning, to stay committed.

One Last Reminder: Empowered action isn't about making huge strides every day; it's about taking consistent, intentional steps forward. Be sure to celebrate every small win, learn from your setbacks, and stay committed to your vision. Keep in mind that the biggest transformations happen when you seize the moment, start where you are, and trust the process. Begin today by taking that first step, no matter how small, and watch your dreams take shape through your dedicated and purposeful actions.

1. **Take the First Step, Not the Perfect One:** Begin from where you are, with the resources you have available. Don't wait for the ideal moment – often, "now" is good enough.

My Journey to Building an Amazon Store

As a testament to the impact of purposeful action and strategic planning, I set out to build my own Amazon store, driven by the goal of achieving financial independence and finding more fulfillment in my career. This path began with a deep-seated desire for change, but it required thoughtful planning, patience, and unwavering dedication.

Starting Point: Research and Learning. My first step was to conduct thorough research. Even today, I strive to constantly learn and grow through new projects.

For hours on end, I've been diving into the world of e-commerce and online selling. I've watched tutorial videos from seasoned sellers on platforms like YouTube and Udemy to learn the best practices. I've read articles, blogs, and forums to gain a deeper understanding of the challenges and opportunities associated with selling on Amazon. I've also evaluated various business models, including private label, dropshipping, and retail arbitrage, to determine which one is the best fit for my resources, interests, and goals.

By analyzing market trends and identifying niche products with high demand and low competition, I established a strong foundation for success. Although my initial efforts might seem small, like watching videos or reading articles, they ultimately paid off. Through these consistent learning moments, I gained a more informed perspective, developed confidence, and avoided costly mistakes.

Breaking it Down into Smaller Steps Instead of trying to launch the whole store at once, I focused on taking manageable steps. These included registering my seller account on Amazon, researching suppliers and reaching out to potential vendors, testing product ideas by ordering samples, creating basic product listings with clear descriptions and high-quality images, and setting up a simple inventory management process. Each step, although it seemed small at the time, contributed to my real progress.

I reminded myself that perfection wasn't necessary; taking imperfect action was more valuable than waiting for everything to be perfect. As I navigated the process, I continually assessed my approach, noting which products sold better and which listings attracted more customers. I adjusted my pricing strategies based on competitor analysis and customer feedback. I improved product descriptions, images, and marketing tactics. This ongoing cycle of learning, experimenting, and refining helped me stay adaptable and motivated. I realized that setbacks, such as slow sales or supplier delays, were normal and vital parts of growth.

The key takeaway is that action takes precedence over perfection. Throughout this journey, I adhered to the fundamental principle that taking action holds greater significance than striving for perfection. No launch is entirely flawless, and delaying progress in anticipation of ideal conditions can result in indefinite postponements. The emphasis was placed on consistent, deliberate steps such as research, planning, testing, and adjustment, which collectively fostered momentum.

Now it's your turn: strategies for success. Whether you're starting a business like mine, changing careers, or chasing a personal passion, the approach is the same: start small, stay committed to learning, be flexible, and don't let imperfections hold you back. Taking action, no matter how small, moves you forward. This case study demonstrates that success isn't about being perfect immediately, but about persevering and being willing to improve continually. Take your next small step today; your future achievements rely on your persistent and purposeful actions.

Visualizing Success: A Mental Rehearsal

Visualization is a powerful tool based on the idea that our minds react to vivid images as if they were real. It's not just daydreaming or wishful thinking, but a deliberate and focused practice that matches your mental state with your goals and aspirations. By imagining yourself achieving your desired outcomes in a vivid way, you create a mental rehearsal, a kind of internal practice that prepares you physically, emotionally, and psychologically for the actions needed to make that success happen.

When you intentionally practice visualization, you engage all your senses and emotions, making the experience feel as real as possible. For instance, if you want to speak confidently in public, you might picture yourself on stage, feeling the podium beneath your hands, hearing applause, seeing a receptive audience, and feeling a deep sense of calm and confidence within. Over time, this mental rehearsal trains your brain to respond with familiarity and ease when you're actually in the situation.

Visualization is supported by scientific evidence. Research indicates that mental imagery engages the same neural pathways as actual physical practice. When one vividly envisions success, the brain begins to develop new responses and enhance confidence. This process helps reduce anxiety, elevate motivation, and prime the subconscious for action.

Practical Steps for Effective Visualization: Set the Stage. Choose a calm, quiet spot with minimal distractions where you can relax completely. Define Your Goal: Be clear about what success means to you, whether it's landing a sale, acing an exam, or achieving a healthier lifestyle. Use All Your Senses: Imagine yourself successfully completing the task. Visualize the details of what you see, hear, feel, smell, and taste. For example, if running a marathon, feel the cold breeze, hear the pounding of your heartbeat, see the finish line, and feel the triumph. Emotional Connection: Feel the emotions associated with your success, excitement, pride, and gratitude. Connecting emotionally makes the visualization more powerful and convincing to your subconscious. Repeat Regularly: Consistency is key.

Engage in daily visualization exercises, preferably in the morning or before retiring for the night, to strengthen your objectives and enhance mental resilience. The advantages of consistent visualization include fostering a positive attitude, diminishing self-doubt, and increasing motivation. This practice converts abstract ambitions into concrete opportunities, thereby clarifying and rendering the journey towards achievement more feasible. Numerous accomplished athletes, entrepreneurs, and leaders advocate for this technique, attributing their success to its efficacy in overcoming fears and maintaining focus on their goals.

Final thoughts: Remember that visualization is not a passive act of wishing for success; it involves actively training the mind to believe in one's potential and to prepare for the journey ahead. By vividly imagining the desired future as if it is already occurring, one creates a mental roadmap that directs actions and invigorates the pursuit of excellence. Incorporate visualization into daily routines and observe its transformative effects on outlook, confidence, and ultimately, reality.

Visualization Exercise: Bringing Your Dream to Life

1. Close your eyes and envisage a peaceful scene: identify a tranquil, comfortable location where you can remain undisturbed. Adopt a seated or reclining position in a relaxed manner. Close your eyes and inhale deeply several times, permitting your mind to become tranquil. When you attain a sense of calm, allocate five minutes to vividly visualize your ideal life.

Envision your environment: What is your current place of residence? Is it a comfortable dwelling, a lively urban area, or a tranquil sanctuary? Consider the specifics such as the hues of the walls, the vista from your window, and the tactile qualities of your furnishings. Allocate your time to purposeful activities: How do you choose to spend your days? Imagine yourself engaged in work or hobbies that inspire enthusiasm, sharing meaningful moments with loved ones, or pursuing activities that fuel your passion.

Connect with your senses: What sounds surround you? Are they the laughter of friends, the sounds of nature, or soft music? What scents fill the air: fresh coffee, blooming flowers, or a familiar aroma? How does your body feel in this space? Is it calm, energized, or focused? Tune in to the emotional tone: How do you feel emotionally? Are you confident, at peace, excited, or grateful? Allow yourself to fully experience these emotions, as if they were happening right now, not in some distant time.

2. Write down your vision with care: Open your eyes and grab a notebook or a note-taking app. Describe everything you see, be as detailed and vivid as possible. Use strong language and sensory

details to bring your future life to life on the page. For example: "I wake up in a bright, airy room with large windows that showcase a breathtaking mountain view."

The aroma of fresh pine and coffee permeates the atmosphere. I extend my limbs, experiencing a sense of vitality and tranquility. My days are characterized by engaging in creative endeavors, engaging in meaningful dialogues, and experiencing tranquil moments of contemplation amidst nature. I am overwhelmed with feelings of gratitude, confidence, and purpose flowing within me. This documentation serves to reinforce the visualization, rendering it more concrete and tangible in your mind.

3. Develop the habit of regularly revisiting your vision: Set aside time each day or week to review and reflect on your written vision and visualization practice. Consider doing this in the morning to start your day off right or at night to reinforce your goals. As you go over your vision, pay attention to any changes in your emotions or thoughts. Use these insights to refine your objectives and stay on track with your broader purpose.

Let your vision guide your decisions: When confronted with difficult choices, inquire of yourself, "Does this decision move me nearer to the life I have envisioned?" Maintain the vitality of your vision: Regularly updating or elaborating on your detailed descriptions ensures your mind remains engaged and enthusiastic about future possibilities. Utilize your vision as a source of motivation: In moments of doubt or challenge, recalling your clear and compelling picture can reaffirm your strengths and the promising future that awaits you.

Final Tip: Consistency is pivotal. The more frequently you engage with your visualization through imagining, describing, and reflecting, the more it becomes an integral element of your subconscious mind. Over time, this exercise will help you achieve your goals, make them feel more attainable, energize your daily actions, and reinforce your belief in your ability to shape your future. Begin today by allocating a few minutes to vividly envision your ideal life, and observe how this practice fosters the transformation of your aspirations into reality with clarity and purpose.

Facing Challenges with Resilience

Changing your life is never a straight shot. Along the way, you'll face obstacles when progress seems slow or even stalled, and uncertainty can be overwhelming. It's normal to feel doubt, frustration, or exhaustion when you hit setbacks. These moments can make you want to give up or wonder if you're on the right path. But it's essential to remember that tough times don't mean you've failed. Instead, challenges show that you're taking a step outside your comfort zone and pushing your growth boundaries.

Every obstacle you face is a tribute to your hard work and willingness to grow. It shows you're actively pursuing something meaningful, so give yourself credit for showing up and pushing through tough times. Embracing Challenges as Opportunities Reframe adversity: See setbacks as valuable lessons, not signs of failure. Ask yourself, "What's this challenge teaching me? How can I become stronger or wiser from this experience?" Practice patience: Real change takes time, and progress may come in small steps. Celebrate these small wins, knowing they contribute to your larger transformation. Build mental resilience: Develop a mindset that accepts setbacks as part of the journey.

In times of adversity, establish composure through breathing exercises, positive affirmations, or recalling previous successes to bolster your resilience. Maintain flexibility: Be prepared to modify your approach if it proves ineffective; occasionally, strategic adjustments can facilitate breakthroughs. Seek support: Remain aware that you are not isolated. Sharing your challenges with trusted friends, mentors, or support groups can provide fresh perspectives and encouragement.

Practical Ways to Conquer Challenges:

- Decompose problems: When faced with a complex issue, partition it into smaller, manageable parts. Tackle each segment sequentially to avoid becoming overwhelmed.

- Concentrate on what you can control. Shift your focus to actions you can influence and let go of worries about things you can't change.

- Learn from setbacks by evaluating what went wrong, identifying lessons learned, and figuring out how to adapt going forward. Every setback is a chance to grow.

- Stick to your routines: Keep up habits that promote your well-being, like exercise, mindfulness, or hobbies. They can bring stability and clarity during tough times.

Be kind to yourself: Practice self-compassion and acknowledge your progress without self-criticism. Remember, resilience comes from persistence, not perfection. Each time you face a challenge and emerge stronger, you're building your confidence and self-understanding. Don't see setbacks as the end of the road; they're just stepping stones that bring you closer to reaching your full potential.

Face challenges with patience and courage, knowing that pushing through tough times is what ultimately leads to real personal growth. Keep moving forward, even when it's hard; your resilience is your greatest strength in building a future filled with growth, strength, and endless possibilities.

Strategies for Overcoming Challenges:

Everyone faces setbacks and obstacles on their path to meaningful growth. It's how you react to these challenges that can turn them into chances for personal and professional growth.

Here are some practical tips to help you bounce back from setbacks with resilience and purpose:

1. Take a Moment to Reflect: When faced with a challenge or setback, it's easy to react right away. But taking a step back and thinking things through can be incredibly helpful. Try to distance yourself from the situation for a bit: Give yourself some emotional space.

Take a moment to breathe deeply: inhale slowly through your nostrils, pause briefly, and then exhale completely. This practice helps reduce tension in your nervous system and clears your mind. Assess the situation: ask yourself, "What just happened? What insights can I gain from this experience?" Adjust your approach: based on your reflections, decide what changes are needed or how to move forward more effectively.

Rejuvenate: use this pause to refocus emotionally, perhaps with a short walk, calming music, or mindfulness exercise, allowing you to face the challenge with clarity and renewed energy.

Plan your next steps strategically by breaking them down into smaller, manageable actions. This way, you'll ensure a deliberate approach rather than reacting impulsively.

2. Embrace Imperfection. Recognize and accept that setbacks and errors are inherent elements of any compelling narrative; your personal story is no exception. Acknowledge your humanity: all individuals encounter difficulties, make mistakes, and confront uncertainty. Perfection is an unattainable goal. Consider setbacks as narrative twists: akin to an engaging novel, unforeseen challenges enhance the depth of your story, offering opportunities for learning, adaptation, and personal growth.

Engage in active learning by reflecting on setbacks, extracting lessons, and continually refining your strategies for future improvement. Each challenge presents a valuable learning opportunity. Adjust your methods as necessary: maintain flexibility in your approach. If a particular strategy proves ineffective, modify your plan, explore alternative tactics, and remain dedicated to your growth.

Embrace your resilience: Acknowledge the strength it takes to face setbacks and come back stronger. With each challenge you conquer, you're building resilience and confidence.

Real-Life Examples of Career Setbacks: If you're turned down for an opportunity, take a moment to think about the feedback you got. Use it to enhance your skills, refine your approach, or explore alternative options. Health or Wellness Challenges: If progress slows down, take a closer look at your routine, get advice from experts, or adjust your goals to fit your current situation.

Relationship challenges: Rather than reacting impulsively, try staying calm by taking a step back, listening closely, and having conversations that are patient and open.

When motivation starts to fade, remember why you initially started. View setbacks as opportunities to learn and grow and be open to adjusting your goals as needed to stay motivated.

Final Reflection: It is essential to acknowledge that resilience is not about avoiding difficulties, but rather about the way one responds to them. By deliberately taking time to reflect and accepting imperfection as an integral aspect of personal development, individuals can transform obstacles into significant catalysts for self-improvement. Each setback presents an opportunity to refine your skills, acquire new knowledge, and emerge stronger. Approaching each challenge with perseverance and adaptability will ultimately foster genuine, transformative success.

Continuous Learning and Growth: A Path to Lifelong Development

Personal and professional development constitutes an ongoing journey that necessitates a sustained dedication to learning, adaptation, and evolution. As I develop my Amazon enterprise, I acknowledge that achievement extends beyond the mastery of tools and techniques; it also encompasses fostering a growth mindset, remaining receptive to new ideas, and persistently broadening my viewpoints.

The Power of Ongoing Learning

As the world continues to change, staying on top of things requires a dynamic approach. To drive innovation and stay ahead, I continually seek new ways to generate passive income, explore innovative business models, and learn from industry leaders. This ongoing quest for knowledge drives my motivation, keeps my approach fresh, and boosts my confidence in my ability to adapt and succeed.

Strategies for Lifelong Learning: Resource Exploration.

Stay current by reading broadly: explore books, industry reports, and relevant blogs in your field. For my Amazon store, I have read literature on e-commerce, supply chain management, and digital marketing, and to this day, I continue to learn and improve myself to discover better ways to understand any business.

Monitor educational videos: Platforms such as YouTube, Udemy, or Coursera offer tutorials and courses on emerging trends and skills. Regular engagement with these resources provides valuable insights and practical tips.

Get involved with supportive communities, such as online forums, social media groups, or local meetups where entrepreneurs and industry experts share their stories, successes, and struggles. These communities offer valuable inspiration, troubleshooting help, and opportunities for collaborative learning.

Develop a Growth Mindset: View challenges as chances to learn and grow, not just problems to be solved. When a product doesn't sell, take a closer look at what went wrong, ask for feedback, and adjust your approach. Focus on celebrating progress and effort, not just the final outcome. Every new skill you pick up or mistake you correct is a step in the right direction. Be open to hearing different viewpoints and taking in feedback. This attitude fosters innovation and resilience.

Test Your Ideas: Strive to apply new concepts in your business or personal projects, and carefully track the results to gauge their effectiveness. Evaluate the effectiveness of various approaches and utilize the feedback to refine your strategies. Create a Cycle of Continuous Improvement: Regularly review your progress, find areas for growth, and adjust your plans accordingly. Look for new skills or insights gained and consider how you're putting them into practice.

The Foundation of Independence Knowledge is a powerful resource that inspires motivation and confidence. It broadens your horizons, strengthens your entrepreneurial independence, and equips you to make informed decisions. Staying curious and committed to learning transforms challenges into opportunities, turning passive hopes into active pursuits.

Final reflection: Achieving success in any endeavor depends on one's willingness to adapt and engage in ongoing learning. By actively exploring resources, adopting new perspectives, and cultivating a growth mindset, individuals establish a solid foundation for ongoing development. The lifelong learning journey is dynamic, exciting, and rewarding, empowering individuals to reach new heights and turn their goals into reality.

Serving as a Source of Inspiration:

As you work toward growth and change, it may feel like a personal and solitary journey, but your impact can reach far beyond yourself. Every step you take, every challenge you confront, and every small victory you celebrate can inspire others, even if they aren't aware of it right away. By pursuing transformation despite obstacles or uncertainty, you create a ripple effect that encourages others to consider their own potential for change.

Spreading a Ripple of Change Takes Courage. Stepping out of your comfort zone or trying something new requires bravery and perseverance. Whether you share your personal stories, struggles, and successes with the world or keep them close to your heart, they can inspire others. By witnessing your resilience, they see that transformation is possible for anyone who's willing to persevere through tough times.

Being a Symbol of Hope: By maintaining determination, you remind others that setbacks are a typical aspect of the journey, not an endpoint, but opportunities for learning and resilience. Your consistent efforts contribute to cultivating a collective mindset that values growth, patience, and perseverance. Each instance in which you select progress over complacency reinforces the notion that aspirations can be realized through diligent effort and conviction.

Practical Ways to Inspire Others: Share Your Story. Open up about your journey, whether through conversations, social media, or everyday interactions, and be honest about your struggles and successes. By being vulnerable, you create a connection that's relatable and trustworthy.

Share your progress openly: Recognize both major accomplishments and small wins. By expressing gratitude and acknowledging your achievements, you inspire others to do the same.

Lead by example: Be true to yourself, make choices that align with your values, and show resilience in daily life. Encourage others by offering direct support or advice, letting them know that setbacks are a natural part of the journey, and stressing the value of staying the course.

Boost Your Confidence and Faith in Yourself

My faith in your abilities, qualities, and potential is unwavering. To inspire others, you need to start by trusting yourself, believing in your capacity to learn, adapt, and succeed.

Developing self-trust means consistently following through on your commitments, even the small ones. It's about honoring your feelings and acknowledging your fears or doubts without letting them dictate your actions.

Celebrating your resilience: Recognize the extent of your progress, acknowledge the hardships you have overcome, and understand how each challenge has fortified your inner conviction. Practicing self-compassion: Approach setbacks with kindness towards yourself, appreciating that growth is a gradual process rather than a linear progression. By fostering this self-trust, you not only enhance your resilience but also serve as an authentic source of inspiration, demonstrating to others that confidence in one's abilities is essential for unlocking one's full potential.

One final reminder: your progress may start quietly, but it's planting seeds of possibility in others' hearts. Keep moving forward, stay true to your path, and remember: every step you take to improve yourself is also clearing a path for others to believe they can do the same. Have faith in your journey, trust in yourself, and continue to be a living example that transformation is possible, one step at a time.

Chapter 13:
Concluding Words of Support

Concluding Words of Support: Embracing Your Unique Journey

As I wrap up this collective reflection, I want to remind you of a simple yet powerful truth: you're never truly alone on your journey. Life's path can feel lonely at times, filled with uncertainty, setbacks, and unexpected obstacles. Trust me, I know that feeling and I know what you're going through, but believe me, nothing can stop you if you put your mind to it. Whether you're dealing with epilepsy, facing personal challenges, or just navigating the ups and downs of daily life, the inner strength you possess is often greater than you realize.

This strength is rooted in your resilience, the quiet, persistent courage that sustains your progress despite challenges. It resides in the small acts of perseverance, in moments when you opt for hope over despair, and in your willingness to reflect, develop, and overcome adversity. Frequently, this resilience exists quietly, providing support even when your awareness of it is faint or distant. Kindly remember: The bravery you have already demonstrated by engaging in reading, reflection, and self-examination at each step of your journey, regardless of its size, serves as a testament to your courage.

Every moment of self-awareness enhances your inner strength, providing you with the confidence and grace to face whatever lies ahead. I encourage you to access that strength, fully acknowledge it, own it, and let it steer you. When life presents obstacles, remember that you possess a resilient spirit capable of overcoming any challenge and transforming it into an opportunity for growth. Use this awareness to inform your actions and decisions. Take deliberate steps toward your goals, confident that your resilience is a superpower.

Supporting Those Around You

It is essential to remember that you are not alone on your journey. You are a fundamental member of a broader community, including

139

family members, friends, healthcare professionals, support groups, and even those whom you have yet to meet personally, who are all prepared and willing to support, listen, and empower you. These connections are not merely words or ideals; they are concrete sources of strength rooted in reality. They serve as a safety net, offering love, understanding, and encouragement during your most critical moments.

Reaching Out Without Feeling Guilty

It can be tough to ask for help; maybe you're worried about putting a burden on others or seeming weak. But let's be clear: seeking support is a sign of strength, not weakness. By sharing your struggles with people you trust, you're giving them the chance to support you better and helping to remind yourself that tough times are a natural part of life. Whether you're opening up about your feelings, asking for advice, or just sharing your story, being vulnerable can create a space for real connection and healing. Don't forget, it's perfectly fine to rely on others your community is there for you because they care.

Love and understanding can be felt in many ways, not just through words. A kind gesture, a shared story that brings new perspective, or a gentle reminder can lift your spirits and give you the strength to keep going. These moments remind you that you're not alone in carrying your burdens, and that the power of human kindness can make your journey easier. By being willing to accept help and be vulnerable, you're also inviting others to grow and heal alongside you each of us connected in this shared experience.

Strength in Community and Connection: Your journey is deeply linked to the paths of others. As people's stories, struggles, and triumphs intersect, a strong and caring community takes shape. By embracing support, you not only improve your own well-being but also help create a space where others feel at ease sharing and growing. Supporting others with encouragement or understanding can be just as powerful, reinforcing that we all rise together.

Practical Ways to Strengthen Your Support System:

Maintain regular contact, even when motivation is low. Sometimes, a simple acknowledgment like "I'm struggling today" can lead to unexpected kindness or helpful advice. Be open about your needs, whether it's listening, practical help, or just companionship in silence. Show appreciation to those who support you; expressing gratitude often strengthens relationships and encourages ongoing mutual care.

Participate in support groups or communities, whether online or local, where collective experiences foster secure environments for connection and comprehension.

Final Reflection:

Your community is a vital source of support. Every conversation, shared story, or act of kindness helps build your resilience. Remember, no one should carry their burdens alone. You're surrounded by love, compassion, and understanding, even when life feels isolating. Lean into this network of support, and let it be a source of strength as you continue to grow, heal, and thrive. Your journey is part of a larger whole woven together through shared struggles and held up by unbreakable bonds of humanity. You're never truly alone.

Embrace every twist, turn, and experience that comes your way

Life's unpredictability is what makes it so extraordinary and deeply personal. The ups and downs, some smooth and gradual, others sharp and tough, are not just random setbacks, but crucial parts of shaping who you are and helping you understand yourself better. Every experience, whether it's a victory or a struggle, teaches you something valuable that adds to your growth.

Each setback imparts lessons of patience, resilience, and humility. Conversely, every victory, regardless of its magnitude, fosters confidence and solidifies one's ability to achieve success. Through these diverse experiences, individuals progressively enhance their self-awareness and acquire insights that will prove valuable in future ventures, relationships, and personal pursuits.

Take a moment to look back on your journey so far. Notice how tough times have quietly, yet powerfully, made you stronger. Think about those moments when fear seemed like too much to handle, maybe during a tough illness, loss, or uncertainty, and yet, you managed to push through. Perhaps it was a small act of self-care, like taking a deep breath, doing something you love, or simply giving yourself permission to rest. Or maybe it was a quiet gesture, a kind word from a friend, a comforting touch, or a sympathetic smile that reminded you you're not alone.

Even the most minute acts of courage or kindness possess the capacity to effect transformation. These represent your unseen victories, subtle battles fought, and triumphed, each contributing to the shaping and expansion of your spirit in ways that may not be immediately perceptible. Over time, these moments accrue, establishing a foundation of strength, patience, and hope that supports you through life's most tumultuous storms. Real-Life Perspective. Perhaps you confronted a challenging health issue, experiencing fear and uncertainty.

Through patience, professional assistance, and gentle self-care, you progressively healed or adapted to your circumstances, each step representing an act of resilience. You may have encountered failure or rejection; however, rather than surrendering, you learned to modify your approach, acquire new skills, or view these experiences as integral to your ongoing growth. Additionally, you might have managed a strained relationship by opting for compassion and understanding rather than anger, thereby enhancing your emotional intelligence.

These moments aren't always loud or flashy, but they're incredibly powerful. They shape who you are, strengthen your spirit, and prepare you for what's ahead. The journey isn't always easy, but each twist and turn adds depth, wisdom, and resilience to your life. My final thought is this: Embrace your journey with gratitude for every twist, turn, and lesson you learn along the way. Trust that the tough times and successes alike are helping you become a wiser, stronger, and more compassionate person.

Remember that your resilience is formed not just by big wins, but also by the small moments of perseverance and self-compassion, quiet, unnoticed victories that slowly build your strong, resilient spirit.

Embrace life with a positive and grateful attitude.

Cultivating a mindset rooted in passion and gratitude constitutes a highly effective approach to strengthening one's connection to one's true purpose and cultivating a sense of fulfillment in daily life. Life entails inevitable fluctuations; however, deliberately concentrating on positive aspects shifts one's perspective from scarcity to abundance, thereby establishing a foundation of resilience and hope. "Start Each Day Intentionally." Each morning, as part of a routine, establish an intentional objective to live purposefully. This need not be elaborate or complex; a straightforward affirmation such as, "Today, I will focus on nurturing my relationships," or "I will be present and savor each moment," or "I will challenge myself to learn something new," suffices.

Please take a few moments: Before commencing your day, pause for a minute or two, breathe deeply, and reaffirm this purpose to yourself. Visualize how you will embody this intent throughout your day. Align your actions by allowing this purpose to influence your decisions, whether it involves reaching out to someone, dedicating time to a preferred activity, or practicing patience and mindfulness. Additionally, consider practicing gratitude daily, as starting your day with such a practice can significantly enhance your outlook. For instance, I often wake up quietly expressing thanks to the universe for the gift of life, the presence of my loved ones, and the lessons learned from challenging experiences.

Acknowledging the small victories also counts: It could be as simple as feeling grateful for successfully completing a morning stretch, enjoying a nourishing breakfast, or simply getting out of bed during a tough day. Be specific: Instead of a generic "I'm grateful," focus on details like "I appreciate the warmth of the sun on my face," or "I'm grateful for a kind word I received yesterday." Small, sincere expressions strengthen your emotional resilience.

The Significance of Gratitude:

Gratitude isn't just a temporary feeling; it's a powerful force that draws more blessings into your life. By focusing on what you have, your health, relationships, and opportunities, you train your brain to notice the good things rather than the things that are missing. Over time, this shift in mindset helps you start seeing the positive side of things, even when you're facing challenges, and builds optimism and resilience.

Here's a real-life example:

If you are having a challenging day, rather than dwelling on setbacks, take a moment to identify three positive aspects, such as your steady breath, a supportive friend, or a moment of calm. Through consistent practice, gratitude and purposeful living become habitual, gradually shifting your default mindset from negativity or scarcity to one of appreciation and hope. This approach does not imply ignoring difficulties; instead, it promotes seeing beyond them and recognizing opportunities for growth in every moment.

Final Thought:

Living with gratitude and intention is not about perfection or perpetual positivity; rather, it involves cultivating a considerate awareness of life's blessings, both significant and modest. By consistently recognizing and appreciating what already exists, one's perspective shifts, turning everyday experiences into opportunities for joy, connection, and growth. Over time, this mindset becomes your innate disposition, grounding you in hope and resilience, and preparing you to confront whatever life offers with an open heart.

Effective Ways to Live a More Engaged Life

Transforming a positive mindset into action that matters means adopting daily habits and taking small, deliberate steps that promote your growth and well-being. Here are some practical and effective ways to help you connect more deeply with life:

1. Cultivate Daily Gratitude: Start each morning and end each night by writing down three things you're thankful for. Begin small and specific: Perhaps you're grateful for the warmth of your morning coffee, the presence of a supportive friend, or the peaceful quiet of your home. Make it a habit: Keep a gratitude journal by your bedside or at your workspace. Use it as a calming reminder or a way to appreciate the good in your life.

Result: Regularly focusing on gratitude changes your emotional responses, making you more resilient to stress and better equipped to handle tough situations. Over time, you'll notice a shift from focusing on what's missing to appreciating what's plentiful.

2. Visualize Your Ideal Self: Take a few minutes each day to vividly imagine your goals and motivations. Create a detailed picture in your mind: Close your eyes and envision your dream life as clearly as possible. Picture yourself wearing clothes that boost your confidence. Feel the ground beneath your feet, hear the sounds around you, birds singing, the hum of a busy city street, or the peaceful sounds of nature.

Use all your senses: Pay attention to the colors around you, the smell of fresh air or your favorite food, and the feel of objects nearby. Connect with your emotions: Feel the joy, pride, calmness, or excitement as if it's happening right now. Let it guide you: Practice this visualization every day, using it as a source of inspiration for your goals and daily actions. For instance, visualizing yourself confidently speaking in meetings can give you the motivation to take small steps towards public speaking.

3. Engage in Incremental, Purposeful Actions: Divide your larger objectives into small, manageable tasks that can be completed daily. Identify a single minor step: perhaps researching a new skill, contacting an old friend, or dedicating merely five minutes to a beloved hobby. Foster momentum: Consistency holds greater significance than volume. Over the course of days and weeks, these small efforts accumulate, enhancing confidence and fostering a sense of achievement.

Here's a real-life example: to boost your fitness, start with a 10-minute walk in the morning, and then gradually increase the time you spend walking. At first, it can be hard, but not impossible.

4. Acknowledge Small Victories. Celebrate each achievement, regardless of how insignificant it may appear. Recognize your efforts: Did you manage to adhere to your routine? Complete a challenging task? Maintain control over your emotions during a stressful situation? Strengthen your confidence: Document these successes, share your progress with trusted friends, or reward yourself with a small treat.

Why it matters: These small victories are the foundation for confidence, resilience, and a growth mindset that help you navigate bigger challenges.

Please be reminded:

Showing respect for others is a key part of living with integrity and compassion. Everyday actions, such as listening without judgment, being kind even when you disagree, and valuing others' views, can strengthen relationships and create a supportive community. In your daily interactions, remember that your words and actions can either uplift or harm. Aim to choose kindness, patience, and understanding, especially when things get tense or frustrating. Also, encourage yourself and others to accept who you are.

Remember, everyone's on their own path, facing different challenges and learning at their own pace. Be kind to yourself when you make mistakes, just as you are to others. Embrace your strengths and acknowledge your weaknesses without dwelling on them. This way, you cultivate a mindset built on compassion and resilience, which helps you handle setbacks with ease and confidence.

Fostering resilience amidst challenges involves cultivating the mental and emotional fortitude necessary to adapt and progress, even in the face of adversity. Consider instances where you encountered difficulties, such as professional setbacks, challenging health diagnoses, or personal losses, and managed to persevere. These experiences exemplify your intrinsic strength. It is essential to acknowledge that setbacks constitute integral aspects of personal development, imparting valuable lessons in patience, problem-solving, and humility.

View every challenge as a chance to grow and develop into someone more adaptable, resilient, and caring. Remember, you have more strength than you think. Deep within you is a remarkable ability to change, be kind, and persevere. Stay true to your principles, your values, and your integrity, and let them be your guiding light through life's ups and downs. Spread positivity by focusing on what you're grateful for, celebrating your successes, and helping others see their potential.

I hold profound respect for each of you.

Chapter 14:
The Man Behind the Scar

There are times when I stand in front of the mirror, looking into the eyes of the person staring back at me. This isn't just about recognition because I know him intimately, perhaps more deeply than I ever expected. The scar on my face remains, serving as a poignant reminder of a traumatic experience I've been through. It represents pain, strength, and survival. But this scar doesn't tell the whole story of my journey, what's beneath the surface of that reflection.

Hidden beneath the surface of my gaze are the untold stories, the quiet strength that emerges in my resilience, and the countless stories that are woven into every breath I take. What it doesn't capture are the raw fears I've faced, the sleepless nights when anxiety eats away at my mind, or the moments when I considered giving up, but instead chose to push forward.

It doesn't reveal the breakthroughs that came out of my chaos, the turmoil of my breakdowns that forced me to face parts of myself I'd rather hide. It doesn't show the nights I cried quietly into my pillow, tears flowing silently as I whispered questions into the darkness about my worth, my existence, and the unfairness of my situation. It leaves out the mornings I woke up with shaking hands and a racing heart; yet, in those moments, I found the strength to whisper words of encouragement: "You've got this," even though uncertainty and my own self-doubt were overwhelming. Let me be completely honest, I'm not a superhero. I'm not invincible.

Let's be honest, I am not invincible. I don't possess a magical shield that safeguards me from life's hardships. I've faced my share of struggles, physical, emotional, and spiritual. I've been broken, overwhelmed by doubts that haunted my days and nights, leaving me questioning the universe: Why me? Why now? I've lain awake in bed, staring at the ceiling, searching for answers, feeling like I was on the brink of a cliff, terrified of falling into the void. One thing I can promise is that I **Never Give Up!** Even during the toughest moments, I always try to keep moving forward. I want the same for you. You got this! Keep moving forward.

Embracing the Journey: A Call to Hope and Strength

Each morning, I start with a simple yet powerful ritual: I look myself in the mirror and softly say, "You've got this." This daily mantra isn't just words; it's an affirmation that carries the weight of every experience I've faced, both the wins that filled me with pride and the losses that pushed me to my limits. It's a reminder that, despite the uncertainty and doubt that often cloud my mind, I'm still here, still fighting, still growing. Let me be clear: I'm not a superhero. I don't have superpowers or wear a cape to shield me from life's challenges.

Throughout my life, I've faced fractures, physical injuries, emotional heartbreaks and failures, and spiritual moments of deep doubt that made me question everything I thought I knew. These fractures have challenged my resolve, pushed my limits, and forced me to confront parts of myself I'd rather ignore. I've spent countless sleepless nights lying awake, staring at the ceiling, feeling the weight of unanswered questions bearing down on me. Why me? Why now? and struggling with a sense of unfairness. Those nights of restless contemplation, tears silently falling, are etched in my memory as some of the most vulnerable yet transformative moments of my life.

During those hours, I clung to a faint hope that things would eventually improve, even if it felt like a distant memory in the darkness. If you're struggling with challenges right now, the crushing feelings, the nagging doubts, the pain - you need to know this: you're not alone. Your struggles are real, your pain is valid, and your journey is uniquely yours. I want to reassure you that every step you take, no matter how small, is part of a bigger story of healing and transformation. Your scars, whether you can see them or not, are a testament to your strength, your resilience, and your ability to keep standing.

Healing is a journey of becoming your best self, not a return to who you once were. It's about embracing the person you're meant to be, even if it's a path that's chaotic, painful, and uncertain. It's about accepting change and growth, even when it's uncomfortable. For me, transformation is more about staying the course and persevering, rather than striving for perfection.

It's about letting go of old fears and beliefs, making space for new strengths to grow, and appreciating the progress you're making, even if it feels slow or hard to notice. Every day, it might mean speaking kindly to yourself when your inner critic is loud, or it could be making that phone call you've been avoiding or taking a walk in nature to clear your mind. Sometimes, it's simply giving yourself a break for setbacks and celebrating even the smallest wins, like getting out of bed when you wanted to give up, or choosing to listen to something uplifting instead of getting caught up in negative thoughts.

Grow with Grace and Gratitude. Remember, every challenge is a chance to learn, grow, and build resilience. When things get chaotic, I remind myself to focus on my values: compassion, patience, and gratitude, and trust that I'm on the right path, even if the path ahead isn't clear. It's about being kind to yourself in tough times, embracing the journey, and recognizing that real change takes time.

Final Message:

If you're in the middle of your struggles, remember this: Your journey of healing and growth is strong and just beginning. Trust in your ability to recover, hold onto hope, and keep moving forward, even if it's just one small step each day. You're capable of more than you realize, and your transformation is happening in ways you might not yet see. Embrace the chaos, cherish your strength, and remember you're not alone in this.

Who am I?

So, who am I? I'm a person who hasn't given in to despair, despite all the challenges. I've faced times when life's burdens felt too much to bear, when my past seemed too heavy to overcome, and when my spirit felt worn down. But I've chosen to keep learning, feeling, and moving forward—slowly, one step at a time. I'm not here to portray an idealized life or claim I'm invincible. Some mornings, getting out of bed feels like a major accomplishment.

My energy, motivation, and hope feel like distant memories, like echoes of a life that was. My body aches, my mind is consumed by worries, and my heart is heavy with fears of failure and feeling insignificant. Some days, just getting out of bed is a win, a quiet reminder of my strength in the face of doubt and exhaustion. But I don't stop there. I get up every day, taking small, fragile steps toward growth. I accept that the path will be tough, with obstacles and setbacks. I stumble and fall sometimes physically, sometimes emotionally, sometimes spiritually.

What really counts is that I find the courage to get back up. Every fall is a learning experience; every setback is a chance to learn more about myself. Instead of yearning for the person I used to be, I've decided to see the present as a chance for growth and transformation. My past struggles, months of pain, nights of tears, and battles with doubt are not scars to be ashamed of, but battle wounds I wear with pride as symbols of my strength. I've learned to turn these hardships into fuel that drives me forward, rather than anchors that hold me back.

Even when I wake up feeling drained, in pain, or overwhelmed with fear, I make a deliberate choice to pursue my purpose. I remind myself that my worth isn't defined by how I feel in tough moments, but by my determination to keep fighting day in and day out, moment by moment. I choose to focus on hope, no matter how faint it may be, because I know that growth requires effort; it's a conscious decision I make repeatedly.

My idea of myself isn't someone standing on top of a mountain, inspiring from afar. Instead, I'm still climbing that mountain; every step is a challenge, and every breath is a victory. As I make small progress, I'm learning that resilience isn't about avoiding pain or struggle; it's about facing the process of rising again, even when the climb is tough and the peaks seem out of reach. And here's the truth: I've come to accept that life will push us to our limits, shake us up, and test our resolve.

But real growth is a conscious choice. Even amid pain, fear, and uncertainty, we each hold the power to forge our own path forward, one difficult step at a time. So, I stand here, imperfect and still healing, knowing that I'm shaping myself through perseverance. I'm a work in progress, not a perfect person, but someone dedicated to growing stronger each day. That's my truth, and I share it in the hope that it reminds you, too, that you have that same strength inside you.

Even when life appears overwhelming or elusive, you possess the ability to make a conscious choice to continue, whether that involves persisting onward, embracing personal growth, or constructing a life founded on resilience. This is because no storm endures indefinitely, and each progressive step, regardless of its magnitude, stands as a testament to your bravery and unwavering spirit.

Built for the Battle

At first glance, you might notice my scars and assume they tell the whole story. But those scars are just the beginning, a first glimpse into a much deeper and more complex story. They're a lasting reminder that life has tried to bring me to my knees and leave me broken. Yet here I am. I'm still standing. I wasn't born for this fight by chance; I was shaped by every decision I made to get back up when I fell, to learn from my mistakes, and to grow stronger in the face of hardship.

Over time, I've come to realize that true greatness isn't about comfort or ease. It's created through struggle, uncertainty, and perseverance. It's formed when no one is there to support you when doubt clouds your vision, progress feels invisible, and the only thing pushing you forward is your refusal to give up. I've had days when I felt overwhelmed by pain, setbacks, or my own expectations. And there have been nights when loneliness crept in, telling me I'd never succeed again.

Nonetheless, even during those challenging periods, I discovered moments of hope an unspoken reassurance that I am more than my difficulties. Occasionally, it was a tranquil moment in the early morning, just prior to dawn, when I resolved simply to continue: "Today, I will try again." Alternatively, it might have been a compassionate remark from a friend, an instant of stillness, or a deliberate breath when circumstances appeared to be falling apart.

Yes, I carry pain. It is an integral part of my story; it is embedded in my flesh as a testament to battles fought and survived. However, alongside this pain, I also harbor a passion for my purpose and for the future I am actively constructing, and an unwavering fire that resonates within my mind and heart: This is not the conclusion. You are still in the process of becoming.

Every setback, every tear, and every moment of self-doubt have made me stronger. I've learned that my true strength isn't about never falling, but about how fiercely I choose to bounce back each time. It's about waking up every morning and deciding that my story isn't finished yet, that I'm still carving my own path even when the journey is hard and uncertain.

What I've learned on this journey is that true growth comes when we face our fears and discomfort head-on. It's in those quiet moments, when no one's watching and progress seems invisible, that our real strength is put to the test. It's in the choices we make to keep moving forward, not because it's easy, but because something deeper drives us. Maybe it's hope, faith, or a fierce love for the people we're committed to serving or supporting.

So, I wear my pain not as a weight, but as a symbol of resilience, a reminder that I'm built for this. My scars tell the stories of battles won, lessons learned, and the unwavering determination to keep moving forward. I'm a warrior, not because I never feel tired, but because I refuse to give up, even when I feel weak. Remember: You're built for the battle too.

Regardless of the difficulties encountered, recognize that your resilience remains genuine, your bravery is irrefutable, and your journey continues. Every stride you take, regardless of its magnitude, demonstrates that you are continually developing. Persist in your efforts. Continue to ascend. Your strength extends beyond mere overcoming; it involves transforming each challenge into the forge that fortifies, enlightens, and renders you unbreakable.

I Am Not a Superhero, But I Am a Warrior

Let's clear the air: I'm not trying to come across as some invincible hero who faces life without a hitch. I'm a human being, flawed, vulnerable, and sometimes drained. I've had days when I felt completely lost when doubts crept in, whispering that I'm not good enough, that my faith falters, my body aches, and my future seems uncertain, even bleak. I've looked in the mirror and wondered if I have what it takes to keep going. Yet, through every twist and turn of this journey, I've discovered a powerful truth: strength isn't about never feeling fear or despair.

It's about showing up, even when those feelings feel like they're suffocating you. You don't need to be fearless to be resilient. You don't have to be perfect or flawless to make significant progress. And you certainly don't have to be whole or completely healed before you can keep moving forward. Real strength comes from struggle. It's the quiet, stubborn refusal to give up when your body and mind are telling you to surrender. It's the courage to take one more step, to breathe deeply in the midst of chaos, and to hold onto hope when everything feels overwhelming.

I have come to understand that those small, seemingly insignificant moments, those profound, life-affirming breaths, constitute acts of defiance against despair. They are instances of clarity that pierce through the noise of doubt and fear.

I cherish these moments. I deeply appreciate the daily victories, the determination needed to get out of bed on tough days, the choice to listen patiently instead of reacting impulsively, and the laughter that unexpectedly bursts out during moments of true happiness. These moments show that even amid pain and hardship, life continues to reveal beauty and resilience. The person I have become is humbled by suffering but driven by a deep sense of purpose. I no longer see my scars as signs of weakness or failure; instead, they stand as proof of survival, symbols of my endurance and growth despite the wounds.

They remind me daily that I stay present, keep striving toward my future, and remain dedicated to a mission greater than myself. This journey has shown me that the most valuable lessons in life come from our struggles, not just our successes. The truth is that resilience isn't about avoiding failure; it's about the resolve to rise each time we fall. It involves finding strength through vulnerability, demonstrating courage in the face of fear, and holding onto hope even in darkness.

If you're feeling overwhelmed right now, know that you're not alone. Every hero's journey involves struggles that others might not see. You already have all the qualities you need: courage, perseverance, and a strong spirit. The path to healing, growth, and transformation can be complicated and messy, but it's real and unique to you. Hold on to the belief that you're capable of more than you think. Celebrate every small win, whether it's a brave decision, a peaceful moment, or a lesson learned from tough times.

These are the building blocks of a resilient spirit, proof that no matter what life throws your way, you're still here, still fighting, still full of purpose. Remember, you don't have to be a hero to be extraordinary. Being human, flawed, vulnerable, and resilient is enough. And in that truth lies your greatest strength, hero, to be extraordinary. Being human, flawed, vulnerable, and resilient is enough. And in that truth lies your greatest strength.

A Heart That Relates

If you're reading this while going through your own struggles, whether physical, mental, or emotional ones that run deep, please know that I see you. I feel your pain, your exhaustion, and your moments of doubt. I've been where you are. You don't need a visible scar to validate your suffering or your strength. Many of us carry invisible burdens, secrets, and wounds that aren't visible to others, but they cut just as deeply.

Maybe it's the weight of anxiety that sits quietly inside us; the pain of loss or grief; the daily fight with depression, addiction, or trauma; or the quiet hurt of feeling misunderstood or disconnected from ourselves. We're all on our own personal, often unpredictable journeys, but despite our differences, we share a common human need: to find purpose amid chaos, to feel connected, and to be truly understood. Sometimes, that means seeking light in the darkest moments when all hope feels lost and the future seems uncertain.

To anyone currently struggling: you are not alone.

Your scars may be concealed behind a courageous façade, hidden beneath a delicate smile, or deeply ingrained within your core. Your wounds could be emotional lingering sorrow, solitude, or unspoken anxieties. They might be mental struggles with anxiety, depression, or intrusive thoughts. Alternatively, they could be spiritual questions that challenge your faith, doubts that obscure your sense of purpose, or a silent quest to discover meaning amidst chaos. Allow me to reaffirm this enduring truth: you are not alone. Regardless of how isolated or overwhelmed you might feel, you are part of a collective tapestry of human experience, each individual confronting silent battles in their own manner.

Don't feel like you have to have everything perfectly in place or pretend to be strong all the time. It's okay to be vulnerable and admit that sometimes life can feel too heavy to handle on your own. What you need to do is show up authentically, faithfully, and with confidence rooted in your own worth. Trust that your genuine self, with all its flaws and scars, is enough to inspire others and create change. There's a lot of power in being real, sharing your truth, embracing your struggles, and moving forward despite them. As someone who genuinely wishes the best for everyone, I want you to hold onto the hope that we can rise together.

When we face challenges head-on, side by side, no obstacle is insurmountable. We can turn our pain into growth, our fears into motivation, and our doubts into a foundation for renewed confidence. Remember, every small step counts, whether it's waking up in the morning, asking for help, or giving yourself permission to feel, cry, or just breathe. Each one makes us a little stronger, a little more resilient. In those tough moments, we realize we're not just fighting for ourselves; we're supporting each other, creating a wave of collective strength that can't be broken.

We're all warriors in this fight, champions in our own right. Our battles shape us, refine us, and prepare us for brighter days ahead. With each step we take in honesty and vulnerability, we grow stronger, more compassionate, and more aware of what it truly means to live with courage. So, let's climb together toward hope, peace, and a brighter tomorrow. Let's embrace the fullness of our human experience, with humility and gratitude, knowing that every hardship faced brings us closer to the person we're meant to become. We're stronger than we think, and together, we'll rise. Remember: You're not alone in this. We're many, united by our courage and resilience. And every day is a chance to move forward together.

Personal Reflection: Honoring My Journey and Inspiring Others

Reflecting on this incredible journey fills me with profound gratitude and humility. Dealing with epilepsy is tough, but it's also been a transformative experience. Every seizure, obstacle, and moment of fear has taught me invaluable lessons about resilience, patience, and the importance of persevering through even the toughest times.

Over time, I've come to realize that our circumstances don't define who we are. Instead, they're just a part of our story - a chapter in a much bigger, more beautiful book. Our story is about the resilience we find within ourselves, the courage to keep moving forward despite obstacles, and the ability to turn adversity into something positive. I've learned that even in our darkest moments, a spark of hope is always waiting to be ignited by our mindset, faith, and commitment to personal growth.

Living with epilepsy has taught me that many limitations are just in our heads. People often feel that certain tasks are impossible due to their condition, but I've found that pushing past these doubts with the right mindset, dedication, and a little courage is within reach. Success isn't about avoiding failure; it's about being able to bounce back after setbacks. This takes self-confidence, even when others try to question our worth.

One key thing I've learned is the value of being grateful. Recognizing all the good things in my life, from my family and health to personal growth and even the tough times I face, has made me who I am. By focusing on what I have instead of what's missing, I can feel more abundant and joyful. Gratitude has become a daily habit for me, and I highly recommend it to everyone. This shift in perspective changes a person's mindset from one of fear to one of confidence.

My goal is to let all readers know that they're not alone in their experiences. Many people face similar challenges, fears, and uncertainties, but these hardships don't determine your future. Every person has incredible potential and the power to turn obstacles into accomplishments. It's crucial to tap into this potential, grow it through hard work and perseverance, and hold onto the belief that better days are ahead.

There's one key message I want to get across: stay committed. You can bounce back, no matter what obstacles or setbacks you face. Your inner light is brighter than you think, and your potential is endless. Keep moving forward, hold on to your faith, and let your brilliance guide the way. Your story is still being written, and I'm excited to see the amazing chapters you'll add.

Sharing my journey, truths, and aspirations has been a true gift. I hope my story inspires you to tap into your own strength, appreciate what makes you unique, and live each day with purpose and enthusiasm. Together, we're lighting our paths, supporting one another, and moving forward with love and resilience.

At the end of the day, you have more control than you think. Don't overlook this fact.

Words of Encouragement to Conclude

Don't forget, your journey is just beginning – it's far from over.

As I wrap up my story, I want to speak directly to your heart: **You're not alone in your struggles.** Whether you're facing epilepsy, another chronic illness, or a hidden battle, you've shown incredible resilience by staying present, connecting with words, and pushing to overcome. This resilience, often overlooked by others, is a powerful part of who you are.

Life often throws unexpected obstacles our way, which can rattle our confidence and make us wonder where we fit in. Over time, I've come to realize something important: **it's not the challenge that defines a person, but how they respond to it.**

Someone is always with you.

When faced with recovery, illness, or adversity, it's common to feel isolated and lonely. But it's essential to remember that family, friends, medical professionals, and others who've gone through similar experiences can offer tremendous support. We may not wear signs saying, "I understand," but our hearts share the same courage. **It's smart to lean on your support system and let them lend a hand.** It's also healthier to tackle this struggle head-on.

When you're feeling lost, uncertain, or emotionally worn out, take a moment to breathe deeply. You don't need to have all the answers. Healing is a journey, not a competition, and it's about the progress you make along the way.

Practical Strategies for Enlightening Your Journey and Reconnecting with Your Inner Strength

Presented here are the strategies and tools that assisted me during my most challenging times. I share them not as directives, but as sincere gifts from one survivor to another.

1. Practice daily gratitude.

When individuals feel that circumstances are worsening, cultivating gratitude helps restore clarity and perspective. It's beneficial to start and end each day by reflecting on three things for which one is grateful, no matter how small they may be. This could include a nourishing meal, a thoughtful gesture, or the resilience to face the day with determination. Over time, this practice effectively reprograms the mind to seek positivity, recognize progress, and foster hope.

Gratitude isn't about pretending things are perfect; it's a show of strength. It says: "Even in the midst of this, I choose joy."

2. See Yourself at Your Most Powerful

Take a few minutes to sit quietly. Close your eyes and imagine the version of yourself that's overcome your current challenges. See that person smiling confidently, pursuing their passions, and moving forward. Feel what it's like to be that person. You're not just picturing someone else – you're connecting with the future you.

What we consistently envision, we make a point to pursue.

3. Make a small step every day.

Don't feel like you have to climb the mountain all at once. It can be as simple as sending an email, staying hydrated, keeping your appointment, or taking some time for yourself. Even these small actions send a powerful message: *I'm still here, I'm still trying, and I haven't given up on myself.*

4. Recognize and Appreciate Small Wins

People might not praise you for just getting up after a tough night, but you've got to push through. When you make a meal, sit up straight, or face your fears, it's time to *acknowledge these accomplishments*. Even if no one else sees them, these victories are a tribute to your unshakeable determination.

5. Cultivate Self-Compassion

You're giving it your all with the resources you have. When faced with setbacks, it's crucial to understand that **healing isn't a straight path**. Be gentle with yourself and have a kind conversation, just as you would with a friend. Don't let perfection be the measure of progress; instead, focus on resilience.

Your voice is the most compassionate one you'll ever need.

6. Tap Into Your Inner Strength

Our greatest strength lies in our ability to bounce back from health issues, emotional struggles, or everyday challenges with resilience. This power isn't reserved for a select few; it's a universal energy within each of us, waiting to be tapped into and used. But how can we tap into this inner well of strength when life feels overwhelming and the world's distractions drown out our inner voice?

7. Shine your light on the world.

Everyone has a unique spark, fueled by their experiences, struggles, accomplishments, and the strength they've gained from tough times. Your story is incredibly valuable because it's your own truth, and it has the power to inspire, heal, and spark change in others. By embracing your light, you demonstrate that hardship doesn't define you; instead, the toughest moments in life often give rise to your brightest moments.

Your narrative shines brightly in the dark.

Picture your story as a lighthouse guiding ships through rough waters. Its light cuts through the darkness, showing the way for those lost in uncertainty or hopelessness. By sharing your experiences through writing, actions, or just being present, you create a ripple effect that reaches far beyond your immediate circle.

Picture a young person getting a diagnosis like yours and struggling with isolation and fear. Connecting with someone who's overcome similar challenges and shown resilience can spark hope within them. Your story can be that guiding light, sending the message, "You're not alone," and "There's a way to heal."

Wishing You Abundance and Unity

Although not everyone will experience epilepsy, many people may struggle with issues like cancer, grief, depression, anxiety, chronic illness, or trauma. Despite our varied life experiences, our common desire for healing, purpose, and peace remains unwavering.

Don't forget that **abundance is your birthright. No matter what challenges you may face, y**ou're entitled to joy, beauty, and fulfillment. We all walk a path that's often clouded by unseen struggles. Ultimately, what truly matters is the journey we share.

Embrace self-love with confidence. Speak with kindness. Imagine the possibilities. Take the time to fully immerse yourself in the healing journey.

Words of Gratitude, Acknowledgment, and Closing Motivation.

My heart is filled with gratitude for joining me on this journey. I truly appreciate how you've welcomed my story, faced challenges head-on, sought out the truth, and fostered hope. It means everything to me that my experiences might help serve a larger purpose. By sharing my truth, I hope others will see their own strength. What started as personal pain has become a way to connect with others, build resilience, and find faith. I wouldn't trade this transformation for anything in the world.

Looking Back on My Journey: A Personal Reflection to Inspire Yours

Upon reflection, I acknowledge a profound spiritual transformation that extends beyond a mere sequence of events. Living with epilepsy has imparted lessons of survival and underscored the significance of **intentional living. It has inspired me to** embrace the complexities, vulnerabilities, and sanctity intrinsic to the human experience.

Each seizure, hospital visit, and tearful prayer has served as a catalyst in my personal journey. I no longer characterize my identity by what I have forfeited; rather, I identify myself through the gains I have acquired: an enhanced sense of empathy, heightened gratitude, a fortified bond with my Creator, and an unshakeable faith in possibilities.

It's become clear to me that **limitations are often just illusions.** Your mind might say, "I can't do it." However, one of the most significant realizations is that *a person's past doesn't define who they are. Instead, it's their choices that shape who they become as they pursue personal growth after those experiences.*

Success isn't about avoiding tough times; it's about bouncing back from adversity again and again. It's based on loving yourself through challenges and having the courage to pursue personal growth and self-discovery.

Gratitude has grown from being just a practice to an essential part of my life. It's the core of who I am, reminding me that we can find beauty even in struggles. It also shows me that there's always something worth noticing, appreciating, and holding onto.

Motivation Prompt

If there is one principal lesson to be derived from this book, it is this:

Always have faith in yourself, even when you feel lost or the path gets rough. It's especially important when it feels like no one else gets you.

Survival wasn't the main goal; you were meant to flourish.

Your journey continues. Your purpose stays strong. And the most inspiring parts of your story are still to be written.

Stay true to your path, hold onto your values, and let your inner light shine, not in spite of your flaws, but *because* of them.

Our world needs your voice, your heart, **and your courage.**

It's an honor to be by your side on this journey, even if it's just through words. May your path be filled with blessings, your spirit stay strong, and your life always shine with the brilliance that's within you.

You have the power to shape what comes next in your life. Make sure it's defined by courage, energy, and beauty.

With profound respect and unwavering solidarity,

Roysan Savinon

www.ingramcontent.com/pod-product-compliance
Lightning Source LLC
Chambersburg PA
CBHW051523120626
46551CB00012B/1050